The
Gi
Bikini
Diet

Dr Clark consults at:
14 Devonshire Place
London
W1G 6HX
Tel: 020 7935 0640

Website: www.promedii.com

The Gi Bikini Diet

DR CHARLES CLARK
& MAUREEN CLARK

Vermilion
LONDON

1 3 5 7 9 10 8 6 4 2

First published in the United Kingdom in 2006 by Vermilion,
an imprint of Ebury Publishing,
Random House UK Ltd
Random House
20 Vauxhall Bridge Road
London SW1V 2SA

Random House Australia (Pty) Limited
20 Alfred Street, Milsons Point, Sydney,
New South Wales 2061, Australia

Random House New Zealand Limited
18 Poland Road, Glenfield,
Auckland 10, New Zealand

Random House (Pty) Limited
Isle of Houghton Corner Boundary Road & Carse O'Gowrie,
Houghton 2198, South Africa

Random House UK Limited Reg. No. 954009
www.randomhouse.co.uk
Papers used by Vermilion are natural, recyclable
products made from wood grown in sustainable forests.

A CIP catalogue record is available for this book from the British Library.

ISBN: 0091912636
ISBN 13: 9780091912635 (from January 2007)

Designed and set by seagulls.net

Printed and bound in Great Britain by
Bookmarque Ltd, Croydon, Surrey

Contents

Acknowledgements

Once again, we thank our children, David and Heather, for patiently (and not-so-patiently) acting as unpaid food tasters for the many recipes included in the book – and more especially for the many recipes which were rejected. Of course, there have been many changes since our children initially accepted this voluntary role several years ago (not that they were given a choice).

David's comments are usually restricted to the token grunt of satisfaction or dissatisfaction which is characteristic of an adolescent male. However, as he somehow manages to consume far more than would seem possible whilst remaining a very muscular athlete, we can reasonably assume that he considers the food to be acceptable.

In Heather's case the situation is quite different. Having spent years as an unpaid food critic for Random House, she finally decided (at the ripe age of 10 years) to enter her school's *Ready Steady Cook*, competition which required planning and execution of a meal within 60 minutes in front of an audience of peers and, much worse, teachers and parents. Amazingly (for everyone except her parents) she passed through the qualifying and semi-final stages to win the final! Well done, Heather! We knew all those years of criticising our efforts would finally reap success.

And, of course, our special thanks to Julia Kellaway and Fiona MacIntyre at Ebury Publishing for their enthusiastic support of our endeavours to improve health through effective diet with this sixth book in the series.

Preface

One of the most important aspects of life for many women is their looks and appearance, and in particular the shape of their body, which is understandable because appearance can determine so much of our lives, from career prospects to relationships. Weight directly affects the way we feel about ourselves, either boosting or deflating our self-confidence, and can literally control our emotions and the way we relate to others. But, even more important than *weight* is *body shape.* Weight is just a convenient measure: *body shape* is the most important feature. And it is body shape that has been virtually impossible to control – until now. Of course, it is possible to slim by simply starving yourself, but on a conventional low-calorie diet the cellulite seems determined to remain on your hips. How many times have you heard female friends complain that they have kept to a very strict diet and worked out regularly but still can't shift the cellulite on hips and thighs? This diet programme will do just that and you will regain the bikini figure that is hiding beneath the cellulite!

The Gi Bikini Diet will change your life. On this programme you will lose weight quickly, easily and painlessly. How quickly depends on how much you are overweight, but you can reasonably expect to lose at least 2–3 kilos (6 lb) in the first two weeks and this will continue until you body reaches its normal weight. You will be eating normal quantities of delicious foods and never be hungry.

This diet is really a lifestyle in which you reprogramme your body to lose weight and your hormones do the work for you. It really is that simple. With the correct advice, anyone can lose weight easily and painlessly.

Introduction

There are probably more books on dieting than virtually any other topic, from low calorie, low carb and low GI, to the more esoteric such as the detox diet, the little black dress diet, the omega diet and even the cabbage soup diet. And most share one particular characteristic – either they don't work for any length of time or they are not geared to the needs and lifestyle of women who want to regain their bikini shape! If they did, there would be no need for any new books on the subject.

So is this book just another attempt to cash in on the craze to lose weight and fit into your bikini this summer (assuming that not many people wear a bikini in winter)?

No, it's not 'just another diet'. The Gi Bikini Diet is actually a medically based weight-loss system that is designed *for women* to lose cellulite from the areas that need to lose it most – the hips and thighs – exactly where you want to lose it, especially if you're wearing a swimsuit.

How can we be so sure that these are the areas targeted for the maximum weight loss from this diet? Simply because the female body naturally deposits fat on the waist and hips first in response to poor diet, and the Gi Bikini Diet medically programmes the body to reverse this trend. We can be sure on a practical level of the effectiveness of this system by following the medical results of our patients over many years. They all lose weight and they are all much healthier as a result.

So this diet is very different from every other diet because it has been specifically developed to cause maximum weight loss from hips and thighs, and it is guaranteed to improve health by including all of the essential nutrients – without much will-power and little restriction on appetite! Surely this is impossible?

Certainly not! Because this system is based on switching off your fat-building hormones and switching on your fat-burning hormones (yes, these do exist) you will lose the fat easily and

smoothly. And if you add the simple 5-minute exercise programme to your daily regime, you will also tone yourself so that
the unsightly cellulite 'dimples' are smoothed away.

The way in which the fat layer covers our body is totally different in women and men. Men deposit fat around the waist but
women deposit fat on hips and thighs in the first instance. This
diet specifically targets the hip/thigh distribution of fat in
women and provides the exercises that will tone the muscles
underneath to promote a smoother, feminine contour.

Everyone who has been on the typical low-calorie or low-fat
diet has experienced the sheer frustration of losing weight from
the wrong places. It just won't move from your hips no matter
how little you eat. This diet is different – *it medically reverses
the process that deposited the fat in the first place!*

A *successful* diet must be:

- Easy to follow
- Tasty and enjoyable
- Satisfying – which means you are not hungry
- Healthy
- And, of course, it must guarantee weight loss!

The Gi Bikini Diet is low in refined carbohydrates but includes
virtually all other foods:

- Poultry
- Fish and shellfish
- Pasta and rice
- Fruit
- Vegetables
- Wholegrains
- Dairy products
- Eggs

Based on medically proven principles, it has been shown to be very effective, not only in achieving easy and sustainable weight loss, but also for long-term health:

- Prevention of diabetes
- Lowering of cholesterol
- Prevention of heart disease
- Lowering blood pressure

Why should you choose this low-GI diet instead of other diets? Simply because it works, it's healthy and it requires virtually no will-power!

Unlike most other diets, this diet is equally suitable for vegetarians, with a varied range of recipes including rice or pasta and an extensive use of vegetables as both main meals and side dishes.

You might also find other benefits in following this diet. In some women it could even help:

- Regularise irregular periods
- Remove facial acne
- Prevent facial hair

This is because many overweight women produce too much insulin – the hormone that regulates fat (see page 9) – and insulin, via a complex process, can indirectly cause irregular periods and the distressing cosmetic appearance of acne and facial hair.

But, first and foremost, the Gi Bikini Diet is exactly what the title says: a diet that will give you a bikini shape and will help you keep that shape for life, and a programme that will energise your life for ever.

Now it's time to find out how much you really need to diet, so check your daily routine in the short questionnaire below to discover your own strengths and weaknesses. Circle the answers that most closely match your lifestyle and add up the final score.

How often do you:

	Every day	Sometimes	Never
Miss breakfast?	3	2	1
Have cereal and/or toast for breakfast?	3	2	1
Buy a snack on the way to work?	3	2	1
Need a mid-morning snack?	3	2	1
Drink more than three cups of coffee?	3	2	1
Have a sandwich/roll/ciabatta/panini for lunch?	3	2	1
Have lunch at your desk?	3	2	1
Have a pub/fast food lunch?	3	2	1
Eat junk food?	3	2	1
Need a sugar fix?	3	2	1
Have a microwave dinner?	3	2	1
Have take-away food?	3	2	1
Drink alcohol?	3	2	1
Smoke?	3	2	1
Eat because of boredom/stress/habit?	3	2	1
Have no vegetables or fruit?	3	2	1
Have no exercise?	3	2	1
Have a very late dinner?	3	2	1
Eat chocolate?	3	2	1
Have fizzy drinks (Coke/Pepsi)?	3	2	1

Now add up the score and check which category describes you.

20–25 You're either perfect or fibbing very seriously.
25–30 Very good. A few problems but a healthy lifestyle.
30–35 Not bad, but lifestyle changes are needed.
35+ Oh dear! You *really* need this diet.

Part I
The Gi
Bikini
Diet

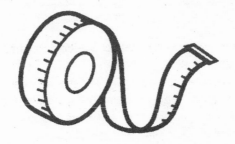

Chapter 1

How the Gi Bikini Diet works

To understand the way in which this diet effectively 'burns' excess body fat, you have to understand how your body 'makes' fat.

The carbohydrate cycle

Carbohydrates are – in simple terms – sugars. They are absorbed quickly, which is the reason why we get a rapid energy boost from a bar of chocolate or a pastry. But – and this is the important part – when our blood sugar levels go up, a hormone called insulin is released, which then starts to lower the blood sugar level very quickly. When the sugar level in our blood goes down rapidly, we feel weak and faint ('hypoglycaemia' is medical speak for low blood sugar), so we have another sweet food to boost our sugar level. Again, we feel better for a while, and then insulin kicks in to lower our blood sugar and make us feel weak once more. And so the cycle goes on. Your body simply can't cope with too much sugar in the diet.

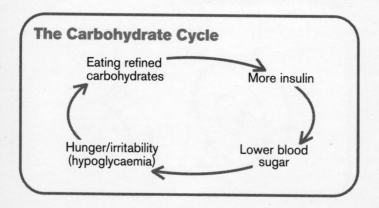

The Carbohydrate Cycle

Eating refined carbohydrates → More insulin → Lower blood sugar → Hunger/irritability (hypoglycaemia) →

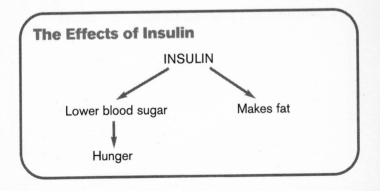

Even worse than the constant ups and downs in energy levels are the difficult mood swings that accompany them. And every time we have another cake or chocolate – which we really must have or suffer the discomfort of low blood sugar, which nobody can ignore we can assure you – the pounds pile on.

Just when you thought it couldn't get worse, it does! Insulin is an essential hormone, but it has one very bad action for the dieter: **it causes excess carbohydrate to be stored as fat**. In other words, it actually makes fat!

Let us go over this again, just to be certain that you fully understand how your body makes fat.

- When you are hungry, you eat carbohydrates, which give you energy.
- Your body makes insulin to lower the blood sugar, but then you feel weak and irritable, so you eat more carbohydrates to make you feel better, which you do for a short time.
- Insulin then turns these calories into fat, especially around the waist, hips and thighs. Even worse, it actually prevents body fat from being used to provide energy, so you can never break down your fat if you have too much insulin.

The Effects of Insulin

INSULIN

Lower blood sugar   Makes fat

Hunger

Breaking the fat cycle

How can you put an end to this vicious circle? If you don't eat, you become weaker and weaker (and more irritable), as you all know. The answer is simple:

Reduce the insulin!

If you reduce your insulin level, your blood glucose levels won't plummet so dramatically, so

- You won't become weak and irritable
- You won't feel the need to eat more carbohydrate for energy
- And you won't build up the fat on your waist, hips and thighs

Even better, if you lower your insulin levels, **your body will start to burn fat**. In other words, you have switched on the body's automatic fat-burning mechanism. Just one small problem. How exactly do you achieve this minor miracle of lowering the insulin level, and therefore converting to 'fat-burning' mode (instead of the usual 'fat-deposit' mode)? Once again, the answer is very simple:

Reduce your intake of high-GI foods!

What are high-GI foods? This will be explained in much more detail on page 12, but they mainly consist of breads, pies, pastries, cakes and confectionery, chocolate, breakfast cereals and beer/lager. Provided you cut out most high-GI foods from your diet, you will:

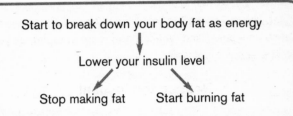

Insulin is controlled by carbohydrates, not fats or proteins, so if you cut down drastically on high-GI foods, your insulin levels reduce naturally, and you start to burn body fat. It really is that easy.

You can now clearly see why previous diets have failed. Almost all diets tell you to *increase* your daily intake of high-GI, refined carbohydrates. Even if you reduce your calorie intake to below the level you need each day, unless you switch off the insulin (and convert to burning body fat) there is always the tendency to make fat. That is what insulin does, and insulin is stimulated by carbohydrates. So you weren't a failure after all; it just was not medically possible to lose weight safely on some of the diets you followed. The system for burning fat was switched off.

Reduce carbohydrates – not calories – to lose weight. Refined carbohydrates are high GI: proteins and fats are low GI.

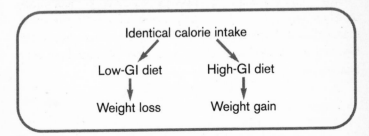

Of course, we certainly do not want to switch off our insulin completely; we need insulin, but our bodies do not need, and were never designed to cope with, large amounts of refined carbohydrates, such as the immense loads of refined sugars and starches in the pre-packaged foods that form the basis of a typical British or American diet. If we cut out the foods that our bodies cannot safely tolerate, insulin production returns to normal, we burn any excess fat and return to our normal shape. You don't see fat animals in nature, because animals don't eat our diet.

Although carbohydrates are a very important factor in the programme, the diet is not actually based on carbohydrates, but rather the Glycaemic Index of foods, which seems complicated but is really very simple.

The Glycaemic Index – the key to low-GI success

Basically the GI is a measure of the effects of any particular food on blood sugar levels.

The standard against which all foods are compared is the absorption of glucose (sugar) and its effects on blood sugar levels over a period of time. Sugars are quickly absorbed from the gut into the bloodstream. Almost all other foods are absorbed more slowly and have a lesser effect on blood sugar levels.

The Glycaemic Index is quite simply a measure of the effects of any other food in elevating blood sugar (glucose) levels compared to glucose.

- Glucose has been given a score of 100 – almost all other foods are lower.
- A high-GI food such as bread has a GI of 70.
- Medium-GI foods – such as apples or oranges – have a GI of 38–40.

- Foods with a low carbohydrate content – which includes most fresh vegetables – also have a low GI.
- Very low-GI foods that contain very little carbohydrate (such as meat, fish, eggs, poultry, cheese, cream, olive oil, avocado, mayonnaise, most nuts and shellfish) have virtually no effect on blood sugar levels and therefore have a GI of zero!

In summary, low-GI foods reduce insulin so **you automatically burn fat on this diet**.

Foods may be categorised as follows:

Low-GI foods
- All animal-based products, including beef, pork, lamb and poultry
- All fish and shellfish
- Eggs
- Cheese
- All 'pure' fats, including oils (such as olive oil) and butter
- Herbs
- Spices
- Most vegetables (except potatoes, parsnips and – to a lesser extent – carrots)
- Low-calorie soft drinks
- Tea
- Artificial sweeteners
- Alcoholic spirits (whisky, gin, brandy)
- Red wine
- Dry white wine

Medium-GI foods

- Most fruits (except banana, mango and pineapple)
- Dairy products (milk, yoghurt, cream)
- Fruit juices
- Pulses (peas, beans, lentils)
- Root vegetables (potatoes, parsnips)
- Medium white wine (for example, Chardonnay)
- Rice (especially Arborio rice)
- Pasta

High-GI foods

- All bread products (including tortillas, wraps, ciabatta and panini)
- All cakes, confectionery, sweets and biscuits
- Chocolate
- All pies and pastries
- Flour
- Jasmine rice
- All cereals (including breakfast cereals)
- Beer, lager, cider, sweet white wine, fortified wines (sherry, port), champagne

The key to successful weight loss is lowering insulin. Reduce your daily carbohydrate intake to 40–50 grams per day, by reducing *refined* carbohydrates. If refined carbohydrates are included in the diet, they must be restricted within the 40–50 gram limit, so choose pasta and rice instead of bread!

Chapter 2 — The golden rules for a successful diet

One of the advantages of this diet is that there are very few rules! Stay low GI and you can enjoy almost limitless amounts of delicious food and lose weight easily.

Now that you understand *how* to eat (and therefore how to diet) you have successfully completed the first step to a successful diet. The beauty of this system is that your body's hormones do the work for you. In other words, your hormones will automatically reduce your weight to the level that is right for you, at the safest rate that is healthy, and then automatically stop. You are not artificially manipulating your body (as on many other diets) – you are simply allowing your hormones to remove the excess body fat *medically*. Obviously you must have a *realistic* body image – waif-like proportions are not normal – but neither is the fat created by a modern diet based on refined carbohydrates. You will lose weight easily by simply following the rules, but you won't lose too much weight on this diet. There is no risk of becoming anorexic. *The Gi Bikini Diet* is based on high-quality foods – unrefined carbohydrates, healthy fats, proteins, vitamins and minerals – and when you reach your correct body weight (and shape) your hormones simply switch off the weight loss process. It seems too good to be true but it isn't. You provide the necessary ingredients, as healthy food, and nature does the rest.

However, before starting any diet or exercise regime you should discuss this with your GP to ensure there are no medical problems that may have to be taken into account. There are obvious situations, such as pregnancy, when dieting is definitely out, but there are also many other medical conditions where dieting may not be safe and which may not be obvious to you. So always obtain you doctor's advice before dieting – or exercising.

Stay low GI

This is the most obvious 'rule' of the diet, but what exactly does this mean? Although there are many tables published showing the GI values of food, the difficulty is that these GI values change as you add together different foods of different GI values. For example, it is impossible to work out the GI value of a meal of chilli con carne, which varies from rice's GI of 58 to that of beef and olive oil which are both 0! But you can easily obtain a reasonably accurate measure of the true GI value from the carbohydrate content of the various ingredients. This is because it is *carbohydrates* that are converted to sugars and therefore it is *carbohydrates alone* that will affect the GI.

Of course, it is not quite as simple as that to calculate the *exact* GI. This depends on many other factors, such as the rate at which the foods are absorbed. But the carb content is definitely the simplest way to keep to low GI in everyday life and so it has been given for all of the recipes in the book. Keep your refined carbs down and you will stay low GI. Ideally you must keep below 50 grams of carbohydrate per day – and definitely less than 60 grams. A single slice of bread is 17 grams of carbohydrate so you can see that the carb limit is strict. Of course, no one is perfect and you are bound to break the rules occasionally but try to always keep below 60 grams per day. There is a set of tables at the end of the book which will help you keep within this limit.

The *advantage* of the diet is that you are enjoying substantial quantities of healthy, delicious food. Your energy levels go up, the cellulite on your hips and thighs goes down and you lose weight easily.

The *disadvantage* is that this is an unforgiving diet. If you go over the 60 gram limit you will automatically start making insulin which will convert the excess calories to fat.

Remember that this is a medically based diet which works by

switching on the fat-burning process we each have in our hormones. By reducing GI intake by cutting out refined carbs, you switch *off* the fat-storage hormones, switch *on* the fat-burning process *and automatically start to lose weight.* But this depends entirely on keeping to low GI because this is the only way to lower your level of insulin, the hormone that makes fat. So there is no possibility of 'cheating' on the diet. Consuming over 60 grams of carbs means weight gain, not loss.

In practice, this means cutting out the really bad refined carbs (breakfast cereals, cakes, biscuits, pies, potato crisps, chips and many frozen ready-meals).

You can enjoy other 'healthier' carbs in moderation. So bread, pasta and rice are included but the amounts are restricted.

Of course, 'healthy' carbs (which are naturally low GI) present in vegetables are included virtually without restriction. The only ones to cut down on for a short time are potatoes and parsnips.

Vary your daily menu

This is the absolute key to a successful GI diet. You can easily enjoy higher-GI meals such as spaghetti Bolognese (carb content 20 grams) or a delicious dessert like crêpe Suzette (carb content 30 grams) by simply mixing these with other meals of lower-GI content.

For example, if you have scrambled eggs with one slice of wholemeal bread (17 grams carbs) for breakfast and smoked salmon with herb mayo and green salad (3 grams carbs) for lunch, you can enjoy spaghetti Bolognese (20 grams carbs) for dinner followed by a dessert of strawberries and cream (10 grams) and still be in your 50 gram limit!

So mix and match your daily menu, and you can enjoy delicious meals and keep low GI.

Include fruit in your diet

All fruit is good for you. Fruits are packed with vitamins, minerals and fibre, and are very high in 'antioxidants', which help protect against heart disease and cancer. But you have to be careful because some fruits have a much higher sugar content than others and therefore a higher GI. These fruit sugars are natural rather than refined, and therefore much healthier than the sugars in cakes and sweets, but insulin cannot tell the difference between one sugar and another so you have to watch the sugar content of different fruits. For example, a banana has a carb content of 31 grams whereas an apple is only 10 grams and 100 grams of strawberries only 8 grams. So watch the sugar content and you can easily include fruit in the diet either as separate pieces of fruit or in delicious desserts such as lemon syllabub (15 grams carbs) or fresh fruit salad with cream (27 grams carbs).

A word of warning! Be careful of fruit juices. These can vary in the sugar content from different manufacturers so always read the label to find out how many carbs they contain. And don't be misled by the term 'natural' fruit juice – some so-called 'natural' fruit juices still have added sugars. For example, a typical value for pure orange juice is about 12 carb grams per 150 ml glass. Some can be much higher so it pays to read the label every time.

Low-calorie soft drinks only

This especially means fizzy drinks, because regular fizzy soft drinks are high in sugar content. Stick to low-calorie (and therefore low-sugar) drinks and you will keep to your diet. Although there is no restriction on low-calorie soft drinks you should be careful not to have too much in your daily diet because some contain caffeine. Too much caffeine on a daily basis is not healthy.

Alcohol

Alcohol is *not* excluded on this diet. (Cheers from crowd!) But it is the *type* of alcohol that you have to watch. For example, a typical pint of beer has 30 grams of carbs. However, a 120 ml glass of dry red wine has only 1 gram! This is because beer contains a lot of sugars as maltose, whereas dry wines and spirits have a much lower sugar content. This seems strange because alcohol is well known to contain a lot of calories, but the calories are not the most important issue on a low-GI diet. Stay low GI and you *won't* stimulate insulin so you *will* lose weight.

We're certainly not suggesting that you should drink copious amounts of alcohol just because it's low GI, but a couple of glasses of red wine, or dry white wine, per day is allowed in the diet. In fact, there is medical evidence to suggest that two glasses of red wine per day actually helps to prevent heart disease, probably because of the antioxidants in red wine. But this does not mean that the more alcohol you drink, the healthier you will be! Any more than two glasses of wine per day and you will be less healthy.

One other point to remember is that alcohol generally increases appetite and affects self-control and therefore if you drink too much you will eat too much and blow your diet for the day.

So what kind of alcohol is allowed, in moderation?

Red wine and dry white wine (such as Sauvignon Blanc) are best. Slightly sweeter white wines (such as Chardonnay) are an absolute maximum of two glasses per day, and sweet wines like sherry or port are out.

All spirits are low GI but be careful of the mixers which should always be low calorie. Ordinary mixers (tonic water, soda water, lemonade, Coke, etc.) are full of sugar so you should always keep to low-cal mixers (which are also low GI).

Of course the same precautions apply to spirits as wines. Because they are low GI it certainly does not mean that you should drink too much. An absolute maximum of two alcoholic drinks per day (and preferably not every day) is essential for effective weight loss.

Some drinks are definitely out on this diet. All beers, lagers, Guinness and cider are out. As are sweet wines and liqueurs.

So not only can you shape up into your bikini, you can relax with a glass of wine in the knowledge that you've not just blown the diet.

Avoid unhealthy refined carbs

How can you tell the difference between 'healthy' carbs and 'unhealthy' carbs?

Quite simply healthy carbs are *pure* foods which have not been refined and are therefore high in nutrients, like fruit and vegetables, pulses and wholegrains.

Unhealthy carbs are present in foods which have had virtually all of the nutrition removed in the refining process, like white bread, white flour, white rice and white pasta. Wholemeal pasta is much healthier than its white equivalent – even though they have the same GI level and carb content.

And the worst carbs of all are those combined with trans fats! These are present in virtually all so-called 'convenience' foods: cakes, pies, pastries, commercial pizza, chips, crisps, biscuits and just about all commercial fast foods (burgers, nuggets, kebabs and deep-fried chicken, to name just a few with outlets on every high street).

Remember, keep to the above simple rules and you will lose weight from your hips and thighs easily.

Chapter **3** The diet in practice

The beauty of this diet is that you don't have to count calories or settle for small portions. It is also a much easier way of losing weight than standard diets: eat as much as you like of some foods, stay low GI, and you will lose weight without really trying! But it will involve a change in the way you think about food. For example, most of us are conditioned to consider high-GI foods as our convenience foods, from cereals and toast with marmalade for breakfast; to pastries or biscuits as a mid-morning snack; sandwiches, paninis and ciabatta at lunchtime; and ready-made meals or take-away pizza as a typical evening meal for those with a hectic lifestyle.

The typical high-GI diet

Breakfast	Mid-morning snack	Lunch	Dinner
Cereal	Pastries	Sandwiches	Ready-made microwaveable meals (with *lots* of rice and pasta)
Toast	Biscuits	Ciabatta	Pizza
Croissants		Panini	Curry
Marmalade		Take-away:	Fish and chips
		Pies	Meat and potatoes
		Chinese	Take-away:
		Indian	Chinese
		Burgers	Indian
		Pizza	Burgers
		Fish and chips	Kebabs
		Baked potato	
		Pub lunch	

These high-GI refined carbs are self-serving: the more you eat, the more they stimulate insulin which rapidly lowers your blood sugar levels; this in turn makes you crave yet more sugar, so you eat more calories, which are then deposited as fat. So you need to stop thinking of high-GI carbs as the 'main event' of your meals, and base your diet instead on lower-GI foods: meat, fish, poultry, vegetables, wholegrains and, to a lesser degree, rice and pasta.

Have a substantial breakfast

How many times have you heard that breakfast is the most impor-tant meal of the day? This is true, but it's also true that you have to eat the right kind of breakfast, especially if you are trying to lose weight. There is no point filling up on a high-GI breakfast such as bread, jam, marmalade, cereal, milk and sugar, because they will stimulate an insulin response, your blood sugar drops within one or two hours, you become hungry and slightly irritable, and eat more high-GI foods (such as biscuits, pastries or cakes) to com-pensate. And therefore the vicious circle continues.

So when you are actively losing weight, you should stick to an absolute maximum of one slice of bread (or equivalent) per day and avoid all breakfast cereals.

Don't worry, you won't starve without cereals for breakfast; in fact, you won't even be hungry. These will be replaced by eggs (fried, boiled, poached, omelette, scrambled), bacon, gammon, cheese, mayonnaise, mushrooms, and fish (especial-ly smoked) … And if eggs or cooked foods are not your taste for breakfast, why not try delicious home-made fruit juices, smoothies, savoury crêpes, porridge or fresh fruit with natural yoghurt. The possibilities are endless! You'll find dozens of mouth-watering breakfast recipes in Part II.

The other reason that you should eat a substantial low-GI breakfast with some fat content is because fats satisfy your hunger and slow the absorption of food. In other words, you will be satisfied after the meal and won't feel hungry for hours – which is exactly what you are trying to achieve.

The only problem is time. Most of us are in too much of a rush to prepare breakfast first thing in the morning. Or so we are indoctrinated to think! In fact, it takes no longer to cook boiled eggs, or scrambled eggs (very easy in a microwave), or porridge, or to do fresh fruit with yoghurt or make a delicious blueberry smoothie than it does to eat polystyrene cereal and toast with marmalade.

For those who are really pressed for time in the morning, continental ham, sliced meats and poultry, cheese and hard-boiled eggs are marvellous. These need not be expensive. Just two to three slices each of pre-packed ham and cheese with a hard-boiled egg (which cooks itself while you are showering) make an excellent 'fast' breakfast. You can prepare fresh fruit juices the night before and porridge takes only a few minutes.

A wide selection of healthy and delicious low-GI breakfasts is given in Chapter 6.

Light bites and working lunches

It is easy to incorporate lunch into the low-GI diet. As different people have different lifestyles, there are several distinct types of lunch to consider: packed lunch, take-away lunch, restaurant lunch and lunch at home. See Chapter 7 for some great low-GI ideas.

Main meals

More substantial lunches, or dinner, allow an almost infinite array of possibilities, from prosciutto and courgette frittata to salmon steaks with lemon butter sauce or spaghetti Bolognese. Meals are no longer based on starchy foods, like paninis or wraps, but rather on nutritious foods such as meat, fish, poultry and vegetables, with delicious sauces to complement the food. There are plenty of great main meals in Chapter 8, and vegetarian options in Chapter 9.

Safe snacks

Snacking between meals will be less of a problem on this diet than it is on others as your hunger will be naturally satisfied by the foods included in this diet – and it is hunger, not just bad habits, that causes you to snack. In other words, your previous diet failures were not your fault: you were simply hungry, and compensated by eating the wrong food. So it really is necessary to have a substantial breakfast as this prepares the body for a successful dieting day.

If you must snack, choose carefully. If you are regularly peckish between meals, you probably need to eat more at mealtimes. Provided you stick to the low-GI limit, you will not gain weight even if the meals are larger.

By far the best in this regard is nuts: virtually all varieties (except pistachios and cashew nuts) are low GI, have substantial amounts of protein, vitamins and minerals, and are very filling. But we can't emphasise enough that it really is better to eat larger meals to prevent the need for snacking.

Other snacks that can be included (in moderation) include:

- One extra piece of fruit per day (obviously not banana, pineapple or mango)
- Melon (4 slices – honeydew or rock melon)
- Yoghurt, which is *both* sugar-free *and* low-fat
- Fresh vegetables (such as chopped carrots, celery, cucumber) with mayo
- Sugar-free jelly
- Low-fat *and* sugar-free ice-cream
- Low-GI nut or chocolate bars, e.g. GoLower products

Shopping: the secret of successful dieting

All the ingredients for this diet can be planned and purchased on just one shopping trip a week. To ensure a successful diet, you must always have the following foods to hand:

- **Herbs and spices** (fresh and dried) These not only taste good, but also have a very high concentration of antioxidants, which are essential for good health. They do not deposit fat and are easily added to recipes to enhance the taste, so they improve both health and flavour at the same time – simply perfect!

  You'll use fresh herbs almost every day, so they won't be wasted. You could also consider growing the herbs yourself, either in your garden or in small pots in the kitchen. Keep a good supply of dried herbs and spices – such as basil, cumin, coriander, turmeric, cinnamon, paprika and chilli – in your store cupboard, too. They can be a little expensive to buy initially, but they last a long time and will enhance countless meals.
- **Garlic** This is one of the healthiest foods known, with high quantities of vitamins and minerals. It is also an excellent source of antioxidants. So unless you really dislike the taste, try to include garlic in your cooking as often as possible. It has been shown to protect against heart disease, cancer and even the ageing process itself through its incredible antioxidant properties.
- **Onions**
- **Fresh vegetables**, especially peppers (red, green and yellow, because they have high vitamin concentrations), carrots, broccoli and spring onions.
- **Extra-virgin olive oil**
- **Fresh ginger root**

- **Cheese(s)**, according to taste.
- **Soured cream**
- **Mayonnaise**
- **Free-range eggs** (large)
- **Fresh beef, poultry, pork or lamb**, according to taste.
- **Fresh fish**
- **Tinned tuna** (preferably in brine)
- **Frozen prawns**
- **Fresh fruit** (especially oranges and lemons)
- **Tomatoes** Try to eat these as often as possible as they contain a powerful antioxidant called lycopene, so stock up on both the fresh and tinned varieties. Plum tomatoes have the highest concentration of lycopene.
- **Black peppercorns**

Other foods that you will need occasionally include:

- **Shellfish**
- **Tomato purée**
- **Dijon mustard**
- **Tomato juice**
- **Arborio rice**
- **Wholemeal pasta**
- **Porridge**
- **Nuts** – virtually any kind, according to personal preference: macadamia, almonds, brazils, walnuts, hazelnuts and *occasionally* cashew and pistachio nuts (as these have a much higher carbohydrate content).
- **Limes**

Remember, these ingredients are replacing items you would normally buy, and not in addition to your usual shopping bill, so the cost factor is not high. These foods will naturally reprogramme your eating habits, so you will begin to require less food without the necessity for either effort or will-power on your part.

Additional recommendations for the diet

The wide variety of foods included without restriction means that the Gi Bikini Diet is very easy to follow: the guidelines are simple and because you won't feel hungry, you are less likely to break your diet. You have a very wide selection of foods that can be included, and Part II provides delicious recipes which are the essence of the diet. Here are a few extra tips to help you:

Vary your menu as much as possible

This is one of the main principles of the diet, as explained in Chapter 2, but it really needs to be emphasised again. You will find the diet easier to stick to if you base your meals on as wide a range of ingredients as possible. Not only are you less likely to get bored (and therefore risk snacking on forbidden foods), but you will also reap greater health benefits. The recipes in Part II of the book have been specially devised to provide as varied a diet as possible. The vegetables have been deliberately selected for their healthy attributes: for example, red peppers contain more than 20 times the vitamin C content of lettuce, and more than 15 times the vitamin A content of green peppers. You can follow the standard dietary advice of eating five portions of any fruit or vegetables per day and still not achieve good nutrition if the fruit and vegetables you choose are not nutritionally balanced. These recipes are specifically designed to ensure excellent nutrition, provided you vary your daily menu. The secret of this diet is that it's not a diet, it's a way of life; if you follow the simple guidelines, you will slim and be healthier – with virtually no effort.

Buy a wok

If you seriously want to lose fat, you need to buy a wok. Although originating in an ancient era, wok cooking is ideally suited to our modern fast-paced lifestyle, as it allows the rapid cooking of tasty and highly nutritious food. And the variety of meals and combinations of ingredients that can be cooked in this way is almost infinite. For some strange reason, wok cooking seems to be ignored in most slimming recipes, and yet it involves cooking for short periods in small amounts of fat – and incorporates 'essential' fats which are vital for health. Heat can destroy vitamins, but wok cooking provides intense heat for a relatively short time, 'searing' meat and vegetables and thereby preserving most of the natural goodness in the food.

By cooking in a wok, you finish with a relatively high volume but a relatively small amount of food, because it has been chopped finely to allow rapid cooking. For example, a carrot, two spring onions, 10 to 12 florets of broccoli, a red and yellow pepper, a clove of garlic, and two slices of ginger root would be sufficient to provide a very substantial and nutritious vegetable dish for two people. The preparation time is ten minutes and cooking time five minutes, with minimal cost.

Get exercising

Regular exercise will complement your diet; not only will it improve your shape and body contour, it will also make you feel much better because regular (simple) exercise improves the blood flow to the tissues of the body, making us look and feel better.

You don't need to spend a fortune on a gym membership, as simple exercises you can do at home – without expensive equipment – will actually achieve a better result. To this end, we have included a simple programme of isometric exercises in Chapter 15. With these you can exercise in the comfort of your own home (in minutes), and achieve the same result as if you had been to the gym for hours. It needs no equipment and no expertise. It also involves no embarrassment. By investing just five minutes per day, four days per week, you will improve the muscle tone beneath the disappearing layer of fat and eliminate the cellulite. If you also walk for 15 minutes three times per week you will improve your cardiovascular health. Of course, all exercise programmes must be approved by your doctor before you start. For more on the benefits of exercise, and a simple exercise programme, turn to page 231.

Measure shape before weight

Use the changes in your *body shape* on this diet as the main criterion of success, rather than weight loss. You will certainly lose weight relatively quickly, but of much more significance is the way your body shape improves. It will not cause the haggard look that accompanies most calorie-controlled diets, because you lose weight without loss of the underlying body protein. You will lose weight smoothly over the body, allowing time for skin elasticity to recover, and therefore without the unsightly folds of excess skin that can occur with crash dieting. So look at your body shape as the diet progresses and watch the way that your clothes fit better, as this is a more effective measure of the diet's success than just weight loss.

Drink at least four large glasses of water per day

Constipation is not a significant problem on the diet, but it can become one if you do not maintain hydration. Drink at least four glasses of water per day – in addition to any other drinks acceptable on the diet – and you should have no problem.

Take a multivitamin supplement

You will not experience vitamin or mineral deficiencies on this nutritious diet (unlike many other diets). However, as a matter of safety, we always advise individuals on any diet to take a multivitamin tablet every day to ensure good health. Provided the tablet includes the daily vitamin C requirement (and most do), you no longer need to have an orange or lemon per day, saving 15 grams of daily carbohydrate intake in the process.

So now you have the knowledge to change your shape (and life) for ever, and actually have more knowledge and understanding of nutrition and health than many so-called experts, it's time for you to begin your new dietary way of life and lose weight permanently.

Chapter 4 Cellulite – the bikini nightmare

What is cellulite and why is it so awful?

In the first place cellulite is just another complex name for fat: lumpy body fat that is deposited in the most obvious places – hips, thighs, waist and buttocks. When it is really bad it also affects the arms and stomach. Just the places you don't want to see fat when you're wearing a swimsuit.

Even worse, cellulite has a horrible 'dimpled' appearance, like orange peel. So it's certainly not the most attractive look. And no matter how much you exercise it just doesn't seem to go away. The reason is that when we build fat it is deposited just under the skin, forming a fat layer between the skin and muscle.

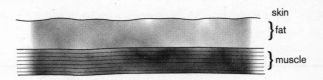

In certain parts of the body – especially over the hips, thighs and buttocks – the skin is attached to the muscle layer below by 'tags' of fibrous tissue, almost like 'strings' tethering the skin to the muscles.

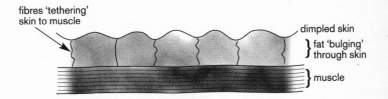

When more and more fat is deposited under the skin in these places, the fat layer grows larger but the 'strings' of fibres tethering the skin to the muscle cannot expand so the fat bulges between the fibres giving the horrible 'dimpled' skin texture. If the skin were smooth, the same amount of fat would not have such an unattractive appearance. Smooth curves can be sexy, but dimpled, crinkly skin – definitely not!

To understand how to get rid of the cellulite you have to understand how it develops in the first place.

Our body deposits the fat in response to too much of the hormone insulin which occurs when we have too many refined carbohydrates in our diet. This process is explained in detail in Chapter 1. Although fat is deposited throughout the body, it is especially deposited over the hips, thighs and bottom in women. And as the fat becomes trapped by the fibrous tissue into compartments, it restricts the blood flow to these areas. Body fluids are trapped in the fat layer causing further swelling of the fat and 'dimpling' of the skin. A vicious circle develops as more fat is trapped. This is obviously an unpleasant situation but it can be reversed medically by diet.

As there is a specific medical process which causes the fat to be deposited on the hips and thighs, *if we reverse that process these are the sites from which the fat will be mobilised first.*

There are other non-dietary factors that influence the deposit of fat as cellulite, such as smoking, too much alcohol and lack of exercise. Less obvious is the relationship between oestrogen and cellulite. Increase in oestrogen levels – frequently associated with taking the oral contraceptive pill or hormone replacement therapy – is often the cause of more cellulite. It's also the reason why cellulite is present in most pregnant women and the reason why it is so difficult to lose the fat after pregnancy.

These all have to be taken into account if you *really* want to get rid of the cellulite.

Of course, there are additional 'fringe' benefits to losing the cellulite. Not only will you *look* much better, you will also *feel* much healthier, with more energy and stamina. As well as the fat disappearing, your body sugar levels will normalise, blood cholesterol decreases and blood pressure reduces naturally – without medication – so you really do feel much, much better. And if that's not enough to make you rush to start your diet, most patients report increased libido, so perhaps you should make sure your partner joins you on the programme!

You can't do anything about the fibrous tags connecting the skin to the muscles. The only effective way to reduce cellulite is by reducing the amount of fat which is trapped between the fibrous tissue and increasing the tone of the underlying muscles to smooth out the skin, replacing the dimpling with a smooth, toned appearance. This is easily achieved by following this diet and increasing your muscle tone by the five-minute-per-day exercise programme described in Chapter 15. (And don't abuse your body with too much tobacco and alcohol!)

Chapter **5** The myths of dieting

Most people have being trying to lose weight in the wrong way for years. Less than 5 per cent of people successfully lose weight by dieting. The problem with the majority of diets is that, without superhuman will-power, you simply can't stick to the diet for a variety of reasons:

- *Hunger* A constant aggravating hunger, with the usual mood swings and irritability caused by low blood sugar, is enough to drive anyone to the nearest fast-food outlet.
- *Preparation time* Hours to prepare – diet fails! How many times have you read 'Preparation time 15 minutes', and two hours later you're still chopping the broccoli?
- *Cost* Dietary ingredients often cost a small fortune. Little wonder that so many people opt for the frozen pizza: nutritionally disastrous, but cheap.
- *Boring repetition* There are only so many ways to prepare a lettuce leaf.
- *Polystyrene taste* A rice cake tastes like a rice cake no matter how many times you try to convince yourself otherwise.

And when (not 'if') the diet fails, we are convinced it must be our fault because, after all, it can't take much will-power to achieve, as we have constant reminders in slimming magazines of 'ordinary' (usually grossly overweight) people who apparently slimmed from 25 to 10 stones without any difficulty at all. So now, not only are we unhappy about our weight and appearance, but we are also guilty about our abject failure to lose weight. What can be so difficult when we have detailed instructions from eminent experts – or even better, the advice of celebrity dieters who seem to lose weight with no problem at all? Of course, the benefits of unlimited free time and money to spend on improving their physical appearance may contribute to their success!

Let us deal with each of these points in turn, because if we can't clear up the mental problem, the physical problem will remain. Most importantly, you have nothing to feel guilty about! You are not a failure, and you are not wrong. These diets are virtually unworkable for almost everybody.

How can this be? We are bombarded with constant information regarding the need to reduce our calories; consume less fat, red meat and eggs; eat more vegetables and fruit, and so on. The list is seemingly endless, and we are told that if we do this we will be slimmer and healthier. This is true up to a point, but the problem is that for the majority of people it is a very difficult eating pattern to implement – and worse, it will not cause loss of body fat in the majority of circumstances.

Losing weight *medically* involves adjusting the balance of the various food groups in the diet, not just reducing calories. Unfortunately, losing weight is not a simple equation whereby if you reduce your intake of food, you will inevitably lose weight. You won't! All experienced dieters will be familiar with the shock and anger of staring at the non-moving bathroom scales, even though they have eaten virtually nothing. It is balance, not quantity, that makes a diet work. And this makes life much easier for everyone, as you can easily keep to a diet when you find food satisfying, and you feel well, especially when there are no restrictions on the quantities of many tasty foods.

In many instances, when you eat less, you lose body protein (especially muscle). So while your body shape may appear smaller, and your waist measurement may decrease, the amount of body fat remains virtually the same. What's more, as the underlying layer of body fat is only slightly reduced, when you give up your starvation diet and resume eating (even moderately), the body proteins are the first to be reformed by the body, so you rapidly increase in weight, because protein is twice as heavy as fat. The classic failed diet! So you see, *you* didn't fail – the diet was doomed to failure from the start.

Now we arrive at the next obvious question: why bother? If all diets are doomed to failure (or involve intense pain and suffering), there doesn't appear to be much point. Well there is! Firstly, *all* diets are not doomed to failure, it is only the way in which the diet is applied that is unworkable. And secondly, you will definitely lose body fat (not just weight, but actually the fat that you really want to lose) on the Gi Bikini Diet – easily, painlessly, with little effort or expense, and even enjoyably. This seems too good to be true, but it is true, as you will see.

For the diet to work you have to understand the real facts of dieting – not the myths. Let us be perfectly clear about this: being overweight is a medical condition, and should be treated as such. Apart from the possible physical problems of obesity (hypertension, heart disease, diabetes, arthritis), the mental distress must be taken seriously: if we are unhappy, our stress levels increase, and that is a real problem for our ultimate health and well-being.

And now to the facts of nutrition. Be sure to read this section carefully – it is quite simple to understand – because if you don't fully grasp the principles of the diet, you won't get it right. The first point to make is that you won't be counting calories any more. You are going to stick to certain rules in choosing foods, which will enable the fat to be 'burned off' by the body. So you will have immense freedom to choose a wide variety of foods in virtually unlimited quantities. For the first time, you will eat well while dieting. Though this might sound like some 'never to be repeated offer', it is based on established medical principles, and does work.

You've probably read some of the following facts before (and almost certainly if you are an experienced dieter) but please read them again, because the subsequent paragraphs will definitely be new to most readers, and form the basis of the diet. Once you understand the principles, you will be able to apply them easily – and successfully.

As most people know, there are five basic food groups that we require: carbohydrates, fats, proteins, vitamins and minerals. The first three (carbohydrates, fats and proteins) give us energy; proteins also provide amino acids, the building blocks of the body. Vitamins and minerals are absolutely essential for the efficient maintenance of body functions (like chemical reactions), but vitamins and minerals do not provide energy, and therefore – provided we ensure our diet is not deficient in these essential elements – vitamins and minerals are not part of the weight-loss equation. So, we are left with carbohydrates, fats and protein. The secret of burning body fat lies in balancing these constituents in the diet.

There are three golden rules that you must understand to diet effectively:

1. Your body does not work like a machine

This is the reason for the failure of low-calorie diets. 1 gram of fat produces about 9 calories, whereas 1 gram of carbohydrate or protein produces about 4 calories. On this basis, you might reasonably assume that fat in your diet (as it has twice as many calories as protein or carbohydrate) has twice as much risk of being deposited as fat in your body.

Wrong! The human body does not function like a machine. By applying medical principles to the way your body processes food, you will be able to eat more calories than someone on a low-calorie diet, and yet you will lose body fat and they will not. Incredible, but true! Now you may begin to see why so many years are wasted counting calories and yet not losing weight.

2. Fats in your diet do not necessarily cause weight gain

In other words, although fat has double the calorie content of carbohydrate or protein, it does not necessarily cause you to put on twice as much weight. If your diet is properly balanced, you can include a moderate (not excessive) amount of fat in your diet and actually lose weight. Once again, this is based upon the fact that the body does not function simply as a machine.

Remember, certain fats are essential for health. (No, we don't mean the bulges over your tummy and hips; we'll get rid of those.) Essential fats make up the outer coating of nerve cells and form the basis of many hormones in the body – including the sex hormones. You can eat certain fats in your diet, and at the same time remove the unsightly bulges of storage fat around your hips and thighs. In other words, not all fats are bad.

3. You can programme your body to burn excess body fat instead of dietary calories

This is the most amazing statement of all – the 'Holy Grail' for all dieters. You can programme your body to burn its own fat – especially from the waist, hip and thigh region – in preference to the food you consume.

How can this be possible? Like most of medicine, it's actually very simple. As explained in Chapter 1, the fat deposited on hips and thighs is controlled by the hormone insulin. Lower the insulin levels and you burn body fat as energy. Enjoy a healthy low-GI diet, insulin levels drop and you start to slim automatically. It's that simple!

Part II
The
Recipes

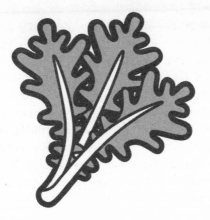

Chapter **6** Start the day

Breakfast is the single most important meal of the day. It prevents mid-morning snacking which is disastrous for any diet. But breakfast doesn't need to take much time or effort and, with choices which vary from porridge and yoghurt to sun-dried tomatoes and herbs bagel or refreshing apple and strawberry appetiser and blueberry milkshake, there is the perfect low-GI breakfast for every taste and preference.

Scrambled eggs

Scrambled eggs are probably better when cooked by the traditional method in a pan. However, this is definitely time-consuming and may not be practical for everyone first thing in the morning. Fortunately, this dish can be quickly cooked by microwave for those who prefer.

For 2   4 large eggs (preferably free-range)
2 tbsp full-cream milk
Freshly ground black pepper
25 grams butter

Traditional method

- *Break the eggs into a mixing bowl, add the milk and a little freshly ground black pepper, and beat gently with a fork to an even consistency.*
- *Melt the butter in a small pan over a low heat and add the eggs. Stir constantly, moving the edges to the middle with a circular motion, for about 2–3 minutes.*
- *Remove from heat when the eggs are no longer runny (but before the eggs have set) to allow the heat of the pan to gently finish the cooking, and serve.*

By microwave

- *Add the beaten eggs to a microwave-safe bowl and place in the centre of the microwave oven. Set oven to high and cook for one minute.*
- *Remove the bowl from microwave, and stir the mixture, bringing the edges to the centre.*
- *Return to the microwave, cook on high for another minute and then stir again.*
- *Repeat the process for another minute, or until the mixture is no longer runny.*

Options

The above is, of course, the very basic recipe for scrambled eggs, and the possibilities for spicing it up are almost endless. Here are some foods that you can add, and continue to lose weight:

- Parma ham, finely chopped
- Smoked salmon, finely chopped
- 50 grams grated cheese: Emmental, Jarlsberg and Gruyère are marvellous in this recipe
- 1 tbsp fresh herbs, chopped finely and added to the mixture. Parsley, chives, basil, dill and tarragon can be added very effectively, either as individual herbs, or combined with the ingredients above
- Button mushrooms, sliced, then lightly fried in a little butter
- Plum tomatoes (two), seeded and diced
- Bacon rasher, diced finely and lightly fried in butter.

*Carbohydrate content per serving: **2–3** grams, depending on added ingredients*

Omelette

For 2   4 large eggs (preferably free-range)
Freshly ground black pepper
Pinch of rock salt
2 tbsp full-cream milk
25 grams butter

- *Whisk the eggs, seasoning and milk with a fork to an even consistency.*
- *Melt the butter in an omelette pan (or small frying pan), tilting the pan to ensure an even coating of butter.*
- *When the butter is hot but not burning, add the egg mixture. Stir the mixture with the fork until the omelette sets, then stop stirring.*
- *Cook the omelette for about another minute, then, using a palette knife, gently lift one edge of the omelette, fold one half over the other and slide the omelette onto a plate.*

Omelettes can be an ideal meal for breakfast, brunch, lunch, dinner, or supper, depending on the occasion and the time available for preparation. They can be as simple or as complicated as you wish. The fillings described for scrambled eggs (such as Parma ham, smoked salmon, cheeses, herbs, tomatoes, mushrooms and bacon) are equally suitable for omelettes.

Carbohydrate content per serving: 2–3 grams (depending on added ingredients)

Poached eggs

Once again, the wonders of modern science allow us to poach eggs either by the traditional method or more rapidly by microwave, which, while it may not seem very trendy, is immensely beneficial to those hard-pressed for time in the morning.

For 2 2 large free-range eggs

Traditional method
- *Heat the water to boiling point in a shallow pan, then reduce the heat to a gentle simmer.*
- *Break each egg individually into a cup, and slide the eggs gently into the boiling water.*
- *Cook for approximately 3–4 minutes, removing the eggs from the water with a perforated spoon when the yolk is evenly coated with a white film and the white has cooked.*
- *Serve on a slice of buttered wholemeal toast.*

By microwave
- *Break each egg individually into the plastic cups specially designed for microwave poaching of eggs.*
- *Pierce the top of the yolks four to five times with a sharp knife, add a teaspoon of cold water and close the sealed top of the cup.*
- *Cook on medium (careful, on high it will explode!) for about 1–2 minutes (depending on the power of the microwave), then allow to stand for another minute before serving.*

*Carbohydrate content per serving: negligible (without toast); **17** grams (with toast)*

Mushrooms on toast

Simple title, simple preparation, but a delicious, rapid and nutritious breakfast. The flavour (but not the nutritional value) can vary dramatically with the type of mushroom used: experiment with various types to discover which flavour you prefer; mushrooms – like fish and cheese – are very much a case of individual preference, but all are equally nutritious, so you simply can't get it wrong. Button mushrooms are particularly useful in dieting as they have the same vitamin content but lower carbohydrate content than other varieties of mushroom.

For 2   150 grams button mushrooms
50 grams butter
1 tbsp chopped chives
1 tbsp chopped basil
Pinch of rock salt
Pinch of paprika (optional)
Freshly ground black pepper
2 slices buttered wholemeal toast

- *Clean the mushrooms by wiping them carefully, and remove the lower half-centimetre from the base of each stalk. Cut the button mushrooms in half lengthways.*
- *Heat the butter in a medium saucepan, and add the mushrooms. Cook for about 2 minutes, stirring frequently, then add the herbs, salt, paprika and pepper. Cook for a further 2 minutes.*
- *Remove the mushroom and herb mixture with a perforated spoon and serve on warm plates with buttered wholemeal toast.*

*Carbohydrate content per serving: **1** gram (**18** grams with toast)*

Toasted cheese

Toasted cheese for breakfast can be served alone or with delicious accompaniments which are relatively inexpensive (in the small quantities involved) and yet quick to prepare and serve.

For 2
2 slices buttered wholemeal bread
Grated cheese (Cheddar, Edam, Gouda, Emmental,
  Gruyère or Jarlsberg)
Freshly ground black pepper

- *Lightly toast one side of a slice of wholemeal bread, then remove from the grill.*
- *Add grated cheese to the non-toasted side and return to the grill until the cheese has melted.*
- *Add some freshly ground black pepper, then serve alone or with a little pickle.*

This meal is limited only by your preference in cheese, because the almost unlimited variety of cheeses can provide a different breakfast every day of the year. Cheddar cheese is excellent for this dish, but for variety try any of the options suggested above. And freshly grated cheese can be mixed with the following additional ingredients before toasting, to provide a truly delicious breakfast (heaven on toast!):
- Parma ham, finely diced
- Plum tomato, diced
- ¼ red pepper, deseeded and diced
- Spring onion, finely chopped
- 1 tbsp chopped fresh chives and basil
- ¼ green chilli, deseeded and finely chopped
- 1 tsp Worcestershire sauce and 2 drops Tabasco sauce
- Finely diced smoked salmon and 1 tsp chopped dill

*Carbohydrate content per serving: **17–18** grams (including the toast)*

Fresh fruit with natural yoghurt

For 2　　1 medium apple, peeled, cored and chopped
　　　　1 medium orange, peeled, deseeded and chopped
　　　　100 grams fresh strawberries
　　　　100 ml natural yoghurt

- *Mix together the chopped apple, orange and strawberries in a medium bowl.*
- *Transfer to breakfast bowls, pour over the yoghurt and serve immediately.*

Carbohydrate content per serving: **19** *grams*

Pancetta and egg crêpes

For 2　　6 crêpes (page 96)
　　　　4 medium free-range eggs
　　　　6 thin slices pancetta
　　　　Freshly ground black pepper
　　　　1 tbsp chopped fresh basil

- *Prepare the crêpes.*
- *Poach (or scramble) the eggs to taste.*

At the same time
- *Grill the pancetta until crispy.*
- *Fold the crêpes into triangles, and place three on each plate. Top with the eggs and crispy pancetta.*
- *Season with freshly ground black pepper, and garnish with chopped fresh basil.*

Carbohydrate content per serving: **18** *grams*

Mushroom and chicken crêpes

For 2   1 tbsp extra-virgin olive oil
100 grams small button mushrooms, halved
   lengthways
6 crêpes (page 96)
15 grams unsalted butter
15 grams plain flour
150 ml full-cream milk
1 tbsp chopped fresh basil
100 grams pre-cooked chicken breast, chopped into
   small cubes
Pinch of rock salt
Freshly ground black pepper

- *Heat the olive oil in a small saucepan, and lightly sauté the mushrooms.*

At the same time
- *Prepare the crêpes.*
- *Melt the butter in a medium saucepan, remove from the heat and stir in the flour. Return to a low heat and gradually blend in the milk.*
- *When the sauce begins to thicken, stir in the mushrooms, chicken and the chopped basil.*
- *Season to taste.*
- *Spoon the mixture evenly over the crêpes, then fold the crêpes in half, and serve immediately.*

*Carbohydrate content per serving: **26** grams*

Breakfast tortilla

For 2   4 large eggs (preferably free-range)
2 tbsp full-cream milk
Freshly ground black pepper
25 grams butter
1 tbsp chopped fresh basil
1 tbsp chopped fresh chives
2 slices Parma ham, chopped finely
Pinch of rock salt
2 medium flour tortillas
Handful of wild rocket leaves
2 small vine-ripened tomatoes, diced

- *Scramble the eggs using either the traditional method, or a microwave oven (pages 38–9).*
- *Stop cooking just before the eggs have fully set, stir in the basil, chives and Parma ham, and season to taste.*

At the same time
- *Wrap the tortillas in aluminium foil, and warm in a hot oven for 1 minute.*
- *Place half of the wild rocket leaves and chopped tomato on each tortilla, top with the scrambled egg mixture, and season with freshly ground black pepper.*
- *Close the tortilla, and serve immediately.*

*Carbohydrate content per serving: **23** grams (including **20** grams for the tortilla)*

Emmental and prosciutto bagel

For 2   1 medium bagel, halved horizontally
6 thin slices Prosciutto ham
75 grams Emmental cheese, sliced thinly
1 tbsp freshly chopped chives
Freshly ground black pepper

- *Lightly toast the bagel halves for no more than 30 seconds.*
- *Top each half with slices of Prosciutto ham then Emmental cheese.*
- *Toast the bagels until the cheese begins to melt.*
- *Sprinkle over the chopped chives, season to taste and serve immediately.*

*Carbohydrate content per serving: **15** grams*

Avocado on toast

For 2   1 medium, ripe Hass avocado (peeled and stone removed), sliced
2 slices wholemeal bread, toasted
1 tsp Worcestershire sauce
Freshly ground black pepper

- *Spread the avocado slices over the toast.*
- *Drizzle over a few drops of Worcestershire sauce and season to taste.*

*Carbohydrate content per serving: **18** grams*

Sun-dried tomatoes and herbs bagel

For 2   4 medium sun-dried tomatoes, sliced thinly
½ tbsp chopped fresh oregano
½ tbsp chopped fresh basil
Freshly ground black pepper
1 medium bagel, halved horizontally
Drizzle of extra-virgin olive oil

- *Mix together the sun-dried tomatoes, oregano and herbs, and season to taste.*
- *Lightly toast the bagel halves for no more than 1 minute.*
- *Top with the tomato and herb mixture, and drizzle over a little extra-virgin olive oil, then serve immediately.*

*Carbohydrate content per serving: **20** grams*

....

Porridge

For 2   400 ml water, boiled
3 tbsp oatmeal
2 tsp granulated sugar (optional)
8 tbsp full-cream milk

- *Pour the water into a medium saucepan, bring to the boil and stir in the oatmeal.*
- *Simmer gently for 20–25 minutes.*
- *Mix in the sugar (optional) and milk and serve immediately.*

*Carbohydrate content per serving: **25** grams (**20** grams without added sugar)*

Char-grilled mushrooms with scrambled eggs

For 2 1 tbsp unsalted butter
1 tbsp Dijon mustard
2 large flat mushrooms
2 large free-range eggs
1 tbsp freshly chopped chives
Freshly ground black pepper

- Melt the butter in a small saucepan and mix in the Dijon mustard.
- Spread the mixture over the mushrooms and grill under a hot grill (no closer than 8–10 cm from the grill) for about 5 minutes.

At the same time
- *Prepare the scrambled eggs.*
- *Place a mushroom in the centre of each plate and top with scrambled eggs.*
- *Garnish with chopped chives and season to taste.*

Carbohydrate content per serving: 3 grams

Grilled apples with pineapple and mint

For 2   2 large Royal Gala apples (or similar, to taste)
25 grams unsalted butter
Pinch of cinnamon
100 grams fresh pineapple, chopped
1 tbsp chopped fresh mint leaves

- *Peel and core the apples, then slice finely, place on a grill tray and dot with butter.*
- *Grill under a medium grill (no closer than 8–10 cm from the grill) for 2–3 minutes, turning once.*
- *Sprinkle over a little cinnamon, spoon the chopped pineapple onto the apples and garnish with fresh mint. Serve immediately.*

*Carbohydrate content per serving: **18** grams*

Refreshing juices

Citrus stinger
Citrus fruits are particularly high in the essential antioxidant vitamin C.

For 2   1 medium grapefruit, peeled
2 medium oranges, peeled
1 tbsp freshly squeezed lime juice
50 ml water (optional)

• *Juice the fruit and blend together.*

*Carbohydrate content per serving: **13** grams*

. . . .

Apple and strawberry appetiser
Apples and strawberries provide our total daily requirements of the antioxidant vitamins A and C.

For 2   1 medium apple
100 grams fresh strawberries
100 ml water (optional)

• *Juice the apple.*
• *Add apple juice to fresh strawberries in a blender, and blend together.*
• *Add water, to taste.*

*Carbohydrate content per serving: **10** grams*

Berry zest

This is the perfect tonic to prevent colds as it is so high in vitamin C.

For 2
100 grams blueberries
100 grams strawberries
1 tbsp freshly squeezed lime juice
100 ml water

- *Blend together the blueberries, strawberries and lime juice.*
- *Dilute to taste.*

*Carbohydrate content per serving: **10** grams*

Raspberry and grapefruit

For 2
150 grams raspberries
1 small grapefruit, segmented and deseeded

- *Juice the raspberries and grapefruit segments and serve immediately.*

*Carbohydrate content per serving: **9** grams*

Carrot and apple

For 2   1 large carrot, peeled, topped and tailed and chopped
1 medium apple, cored and chopped
1 tsp orange zest

- *Juice the carrot, apple and orange zest and serve immediately.*

*Carbohydrate content per serving: **8** grams*

....

Strawberry and blackberry

For 2   100 grams strawberries
100 grams blackberries

- *Juice the berries and serve immediately.*

*Carbohydrate content per serving: **9** grams*

....

Avocado, tomato and basil

For 2   1 small Hass avocado, stone removed, peeled and chopped
3 medium plum tomatoes on the vine, chopped
6–8 large basil leaves, washed and finely chopped

- *Blend the ingredients and serve immediately.*

*Carbohydrate content per serving: **4** grams*

Smoothies

Mango and strawberry milkshake
This contains vitamins A and C from the fruits, and calcium and vitamin D from the milk.

For 2   1 mango
           100 grams ripe strawberries
           125 ml cold full-cream milk

- *Juice the mango.*
- *Blend together the mango juice, strawberries and milk.*

*Carbohydrate content per serving: **14 grams***

Blueberry milkshake
Once again, a perfect combination of vitamin C from the fruit, and calcium and vitamin D from milk.

For 2   150 grams fresh blueberries
           200 ml cold full-cream milk

- *Juice the blueberries.*
- *Blend with the milk.*

*Carbohydrate content per serving: **16 grams***

Mint and cucumber

For 2   1 tbsp chopped mint leaves
1 medium English cucumber, peeled, deseeded and
  chopped
200 ml natural yoghurt

- *Blend together the mint, cucumber and yoghurt and
serve immediately.*

*Carbohydrate content per serving: **12** grams*

Raspberry and orange

For 2   100 grams raspberries
100 ml natural yoghurt
100 ml freshly squeezed orange juice

- *Blend together the raspberries and yoghurt.*
- *Add the orange juice, blend until smooth and serve
immediately.*

*Carbohydrate content per serving: **9** grams*

Berry surprise

For 2   100 grams blackberries
100 grams blueberries
100 ml natural yoghurt, chilled
Crushed ice

- *Blend together the blackberries, blueberries, yoghurt
and ice, and serve immediately.*

*Carbohydrate content per serving: **16** grams*

Chapter **7** Lunch-on-the-run

For most of us lunch is usually a quick sandwich or panini either at the office or at home. The secret of successful dieting is variety. The GI Bikini Diet is perfect in this respect because so many delicious foods are included. Enjoy a barbecue turkey salad one day and spinach and Emmental crêpes the next. Or prepare a quick-and-easy carrot and coriander soup the previous evening and microwave at work!

Soups

Chilled cucumber soup

For 2   1 large cucumber, peeled and diced
400 ml vegetable stock
1½ tbsp chopped fresh chives
Pinch of sea salt
Freshly ground black pepper
100 ml single cream

- *Add the cucumber to the stock in a large saucepan, bring to the boil, then reduce the heat and simmer gently for 30 minutes.*
- *Stir in a tbsp of chopped fresh chives, season to taste and purée.*
- *Return the puréed soup to the pan, stir in the cream and heat through gently for about 4–5 minutes.*
- *Chill in the fridge for 2 hours then serve, garnished with the remaining chopped chives.*

*Carbohydrate content per serving: **16** grams*

Gazpacho

For 2   1 medium red pepper, deseeded and chopped
1 medium green pepper, deseeded and chopped
1 large green chilli, deseeded and finely chopped
1 garlic clove, peeled and finely chopped
1 Lebanese cucumber, chopped
1 medium red onion, peeled and chopped
400 grams ripe plum tomatoes, peeled and chopped
2 tbsp red wine vinegar
3 tbsp extra-virgin olive oil
300 ml unsweetened tomato juice
2 tsp chopped fresh basil
Pinch of rock salt
Freshly ground black pepper

- *Before commencing, set aside a little of the chopped red and green peppers, cucumber, onion and chilli – sufficient for garnish later.*
- *Blend the peppers, cucumber, onion, chilli, garlic, tomatoes, red wine vinegar, olive oil and tomato juice in a food processor.*
- *Season to taste and chill for at least 2 hours in the fridge.*
- *Serve chilled, garnished with the chopped peppers, cucumber, onion and red chilli.*

Carbohydrate content per serving: **27** *grams*

Tomato and basil soup

For 2 2 tbsp extra-virgin olive oil

350 grams plum tomatoes, peeled and chopped

1 garlic clove, peeled and finely chopped

3 spring onions, finely chopped

2 tbsp chopped fresh basil

1 bay leaf

350 ml chicken (or vegetable) stock

1 tbsp tomato purée

Freshly ground black pepper

2 tsp cornflour

100 ml single cream

Pinch of rock salt

2 tsp chopped fresh basil, to garnish

A simple method of peeling tomatoes is to cut a shallow cross through the skin of each tomato at its base. Place the tomatoes in a bowl of boiling water for 30 seconds, then drain off the boiling water. Immerse the tomatoes in cold water for a few seconds, then the skin should peel easily. Ripe tomatoes are much easier to peel.

- *Heat the olive oil in a large saucepan, then add the tomatoes, garlic and spring onions, and cook for 2–3 minutes, stirring frequently.*
- *Add the basil, bay leaf, stock and tomato purée. Season with freshly ground black pepper, but do not add further salt at this stage as the stock may be quite salty.*
- *Bring to the boil and simmer for 20–30 minutes, then sieve the mixture into a clean saucepan.*
- *Mix the cornflour with a little cold water to make a smooth paste and add to the soup, mixing evenly. Stir over a low heat until the soup thickens.*

- *Add salt to taste (although none may be necessary).*
- *Stir in the cream and serve garnished with chopped basil.*

*Carbohydrate content per serving: **20** grams*

• •

Carrot and coriander soup

For 2
2 tbsp extra-virgin olive oil
1 medium onion, peeled and finely diced
1 garlic clove, peeled and finely chopped
200 grams carrots, finely grated
400 ml chicken stock
1 tbsp chopped fresh coriander
2 tsp freshly squeezed lemon juice
Pinch of rock salt (optional)
Freshly ground black pepper
100 ml single cream
2 tsp chopped fresh chives, to garnish

- *Heat the olive oil in a medium saucepan and sauté the onion and garlic for about a minute.*
- *Add the carrots, mixing well, and sauté on a very low heat for 6–8 minutes.*
- *Stir in the chicken stock and coriander. Add the lemon juice, season to taste and simmer for 25–30 minutes. (This soup can be puréed; however, we prefer the chunky variety.)*
- *Stir in the cream and serve immediately, garnished with chopped chives.*

*Carbohydrate content per serving: **9** grams*

Lemon and chicken soup

Lemon and chicken are a perfect gastronomic combination.
The sharpness of the lemon is absorbed to perfection by the
texture of the chicken. Apart from providing all of our essential
amino acids from chicken, this recipe is also a rich source of
the powerful antioxidants vitamin C from lemon juice and
vitamin A from carrots.

For 2
30 grams unsalted butter
1 medium brown onion, peeled and diced
1 medium carrot, peeled and grated
1 large ready-cooked chicken breast (approx
150 grams), chopped
3 tbsp freshly squeezed lemon juice
1 bay leaf
400 ml chicken stock
1 tbsp dry sherry
Pinch of rock salt
Freshly ground black pepper
100 ml single cream

- *Melt the butter in a large saucepan and gently sauté the onion and carrot for 2–3 minutes.*
- *Add the chicken, lemon juice, bay leaf, stock and sherry, and season to taste.*
- *Bring to the boil, then reduce the heat and simmer gently for about 45 minutes.*
- *Remove the bay leaf, and purée the soup in a food processor.*
- *Stir in about 80 ml of cream and heat through gently.*
- *Serve immediately with a swirl of cream.*

Carbohydrate content per serving: **8 grams**

Creamy mushroom soup

For 2   1 tbsp extra-virgin olive oil
2 shallots, peeled and finely chopped
1 garlic clove, peeled and finely chopped
60 grams button mushrooms, wiped and finely sliced
½ tbsp plain flour
150 ml chicken (or vegetable) stock
150 ml full-cream milk
Pinch of salt
Freshly ground black pepper
1 tbsp medium sherry (or Marsala)
1 tbsp freshly chopped flat-leaf parsley, to garnish

- *Heat the extra-virgin olive oil in a medium saucepan and gently sauté the shallots and garlic for 2–3 minutes.*
- *Stir in the mushrooms and cook for a further 2–3 minutes.*
- *Remove from the heat and stir in the flour.*
- *Return to a gentle heat and stir in the stock and milk.*
- *Season to taste then simmer gently for 2–3 minutes, but do not allow to boil.*
- *Purée the soup.*
- *Stir in the medium sherry (or Marsala) and serve immediately, garnished with freshly chopped flat-leaf parsley.*

*Carbohydrate content per serving: **12** grams*

Tofu and red pepper soup

For 2   450 ml vegetable stock
2 slices fresh ginger root, peeled and grated
100 grams tofu, chopped into 2 cm cubes
1 small red pepper, deseeded and finely sliced
50 grams bamboo shoots, drained and finely sliced
2 spring onions, chopped into 1–2 cm lengths on the
    diagonal
Pinch of sea salt
Freshly ground black pepper
½ tbsp freshly chopped coriander leaves

- *Bring the vegetable stock to the boil, then add the
  ginger, tofu, red pepper, bamboo shoots and spring
  onions.*
- *Season to taste and simmer gently for 15 minutes.*
- *Serve immediately and sprinkle over freshly chopped
  coriander leaves.*

Carbohydrate content per serving: **11** *grams*

Sandwiches

In sandwiches or toast, always try to use wholemeal bread, rather than white or brown. Wholemeal bread is rich in vitamin B, and actually slows the digestive process, which is an essential part of healthy nutrition as it allows our body to absorb the nutrients from the food.

Avocado

For 2
1 small ripe Hass avocado, halved, peeled, stoned and finely sliced with either diced plum tomato or sliced mozzarella cheese, or both
2 slices buttered wholemeal bread
1 tbsp extra-virgin olive oil
2 tsp balsamic vinegar
Freshly ground black pepper

- *Arrange the sliced avocado on a slice of buttered wholemeal bread.*
- *Top with either diced plum tomato or sliced mozzarella cheese (or both).*
- *Drizzle the extra-virgin olive oil and balsamic vinegar over the filling and season with freshly ground black pepper.*

Carbohydrate content per serving: 3 grams (20 grams with bread)

Egg mayonnaise

Probably the easiest way to prepare eggs for sandwiches is by hard-boiling them at breakfast, then cooling them and chopping them finely. They can be used in an almost unlimited range of combinations. A brief selection of possibilities follows.

For 2   3 large free-range eggs, hard-boiled and chopped
         1 tbsp mayonnaise, home-made (page 210) or
            commercial
         Freshly ground black pepper
         2 slices buttered wholemeal bread

- *Mix the eggs with mayonnaise, season with freshly ground black pepper and serve on buttered wholemeal bread.*

*Carbohydrate content per serving: **17** grams (i.e. the carbohydrate content of the bread; eggs and mayonnaise are virtually carbohydrate-free)*

This basic recipe can be enhanced by the following additions:

- diced avocado
- finely chopped vine-ripened tomato
- sliced smoked salmon
- chopped fresh basil
- sliced Lebanese cucumber and chopped fresh chives
- curly endive lettuce and chopped fresh coriander
- red and yellow peppers, deseeded and finely diced
- diced vine-ripened tomatoes with chopped fresh chives and basil
- diced green chilli and avocado

*Carbohydrate content per serving: **2–3** grams*

Chicken with mayonnaise and avocado

For 2
1 small chicken breast fillet
2 tbsp extra-virgin olive oil
1 tbsp mayonnaise (page 210)
Half a small ripe Hass avocado, finely sliced
2 slices buttered wholemeal bread
Freshly ground black pepper

- *Sauté the chicken fillet in the olive oil for approximately 5 minutes on each side, turning once, until cooked. Set aside to cool, then slice finely.*
- *Mix with the mayonnaise and spoon on to a slice of buttered wholemeal bread.*
- *Arrange the avocado slices on the chicken and season with freshly ground black pepper.*

Carbohydrate content per serving: 1 gram (18 grams with bread)

Prawn mayonnaise open sandwich

For 2
150 grams cooked prawns
1 tbsp mayonnaise (page 210)
2 spring onions, finely chopped
2 slices buttered wholemeal bread
Freshly ground black pepper

- *Mix together the prawns, mayonnaise and chopped spring onions.*
- *Spoon the mixture on to two slices of buttered wholemeal bread.*
- *Season to taste with freshly ground black pepper.*

Carbohydrate content per serving: 18 grams (1 gram without bread)

Tuna mayonnaise open sandwich

We suggest using tuna in brine or springwater – not to avoid the oil, but because tuna in brine is easily drained and can then absorb the flavours of mayonnaise and other additives more easily.

For 2   200 gram tin tuna (in brine or springwater), drained
1 tbsp mayonnaise (page 210)
1 tbsp chopped fresh basil
1 tsp chopped fresh coriander
Freshly ground black pepper
2 slices buttered wholemeal bread
1 vine-ripened tomato, diced (optional)
½ small red pepper, deseeded and sliced thinly
(optional)
1 tsp chopped fresh chives

- *Flake the tuna and mix with 1 tbsp mayonnaise, chopped basil and coriander, and freshly ground black pepper.*
- *Spoon the mixture liberally on two slices of buttered wholemeal bread.*
- *Top with diced vine-ripened tomato (and/or sliced red pepper with chopped fresh chives).*

*Carbohydrate content per serving: **19** grams (**2** grams without bread)*

Bacon, lettuce and tomato open sandwich

For 2   4 rashers cooked bacon
Small handful of mixed lettuce leaves (frisée, mizuna, green oak, rocket)
2 slices buttered wholemeal bread (or toast)
2 medium plum tomatoes (preferably on the vine), sliced
Drizzle of Worcestershire sauce, to taste (optional)
Freshly ground black pepper

- *Cook the bacon, either fry, grill or by microwave.*
- *Arrange the mixed lettuce leaves on the buttered wholemeal bread (or toast, if preferred).*
- *Top with tomato slices and cooked bacon rashers.*
- *Drizzle over a few drops of Worcestershire sauce (optional) and season to taste with freshly ground black pepper.*

Carbohydrate content per serving: 19 grams (only 2 grams without bread)

Salads and pâtés

Roasted pepper and Bocconcini salad
If possible, try to use the true Bocconcini, made from buffalo milk. The difference in taste is well worth the effort!

For 2
1 medium yellow pepper, deseeded and quartered
1 medium red pepper, deseeded and quartered
2 tbsp extra-virgin olive oil
100 grams Bocconcini cheese, thinly sliced
2 medium vine-ripened tomatoes, sliced
Pinch of rock salt
Freshly ground black pepper
Balsamic vinaigrette (page 208)
Fresh basil leaves, to garnish

* *Place the peppers in an oven-safe dish, drizzle over the extra-virgin olive oil, cover with pierced aluminium foil and bake in the centre of a pre-heated oven at 180°C (gas mark 4) for 20–25 minutes.*
* *Remove from the oven and set aside. When cool, slice into thin strips.*
* *Mix together the peppers and place in the centre of the plates.*
* *Arrange the tomato and Bocconcini slices alternately around the peppers, season to taste, drizzle over the balsamic vinaigrette and garnish with fresh basil leaves.*

*Carbohydrate content per serving: **8** grams*

Semi-dried tomatoes with herbs
Tomatoes and thyme are foods with an extremely high concentration of antioxidants.

For 4   8 large plum tomatoes, quartered lengthways
1 tbsp chopped fresh basil
1 tbsp chopped fresh thyme
Freshly ground black pepper
2 tbsp extra-virgin olive oil

- *Place the tomatoes skin down on a wire rack in a baking tray, sprinkle with the herbs and pepper, and cook in the centre of a pre-heated oven at 150°C (gas mark 2) for about 2½–3 hours.*
- *Remove from the oven and set aside to cool.*
- *Mix with extra-virgin olive oil, and cool in the fridge for 3–4 hours before use.*

*Carbohydrate content per serving: **6** grams*

Cherry tomatoes with basil and coriander
For 2   50 grams unsalted butter
10 cherry vine tomatoes
1 tsp chopped fresh basil
1 tsp chopped fresh coriander
Freshly ground black pepper

- *Heat the butter in a medium saucepan, add the cherry tomatoes, basil and coriander and sauté for 2–3 minutes.*
- *Season to taste with freshly ground black pepper and serve immediately.*

*Carbohydrate content per serving: **4** grams*

Scallop and calamari salad

Shellfish are such a healthy food, why restrict yourself to only one! The flavours of different shellfish merge beautifully together, and are particularly enhanced by garlic and ginger. This recipe provides an excellent source of iron, and all the essential amino acids.

For 2
- 30 grams butter
- 4 large scallops
- 2 tbsp extra-virgin olive oil
- 1 tsp sesame oil
- 2 garlic cloves, peeled and chopped finely
- 2 slices fresh ginger root, peeled and chopped finely
- 8 raw tiger prawns, peeled and deveined (tails on)
- 200 grams fresh calamari tubes, chopped into 1 cm rings
- 100 grams mixed wild rocket and red oak lettuce
- 4 spring onions, finely chopped
- 1 tbsp chopped fresh coriander
- Freshly ground black pepper
- Oriental vinaigrette (page 207)
- Lime wedges

- *Melt the butter in a small saucepan.*
- *Separate the corals from the scallops, slice the scallops into rounds horizontally and gently sauté the scallops and corals for 3–4 minutes.*
- *Remove them from the pan with a perforated spoon, cover and set aside.*
- *Heat the olive oil and sesame oil in a wok and sauté the garlic and ginger for a minute.*
- *Add the prawns and calamari, and stir-fry for 2–3 minutes.*

- *Add the cooked scallops and heat through gently for about a minute.*
- *Toss the wild rocket, red oak lettuce, spring onions and coriander, season to taste and transfer to plates.*
- *Arrange the scallops, prawns and calamari on the salad, drizzle over the dressing, and serve with lime wedges.*

Carbohydrate content per serving: negligible

....

Feta and olive salad
This is often described as a Greek salad, but is actually present in many Mediterranean countries.

For 2
2 large plum tomatoes, quartered lengthways
1 Lebanese cucumber, chopped on the diagonal
3 spring onions, chopped into 3–4 cm lengths on the diagonal
100 grams black olives, halved and stoned
100 grams Feta cheese, cubed
Freshly ground black pepper
French vinaigrette (page 206) or lemon and coriander vinaigrette (page 208)

- *Mix together the ingredients of the salad, and dress with either a simple vinaigrette, or lemon and coriander vinaigrette for extra zest.*

*Carbohydrate content per serving: **5** grams*

Chilli beef salad

Strange though it may seem, you can actually omit the chilli in this recipe, without losing the taste. So if you don't like spicy flavours, leave out the chilli! It still tastes delicious, and is very healthy and nutritious.

For 2
250 grams lean beef fillet
150 grams mixed crispy lettuce leaves (curly endive, coral, green oak leaf, and mizuna) and rocket
1 medium Lebanese cucumber, sliced lengthways
Fresh coriander leaves, to garnish

Marinade
1 tbsp oyster sauce
1 tbsp sweet sherry
1 tbsp extra-virgin olive oil
2 slices fresh ginger root, peeled and finely chopped
1 garlic clove, peeled and finely chopped
Freshly ground black pepper

Dressing
4 tbsp extra-virgin olive oil
1 tbsp chopped fresh basil leaves
1 tbsp white wine vinegar
1 small red chilli, deseeded and chopped (optional)
1 spring onion, finely chopped
1 stalk lemon grass, outer leaves removed, finely chopped
Juice of a freshly squeezed lemon
Pinch of rock salt
Freshly ground black pepper

- *Mix together the ingredients of the marinade, and marinate the beef for 4–6 hours.*
- *Place the beef in a roasting tin, pour over the marinade and cover.*
- *Cook in the centre of a pre-heated oven at 200°C (gas mark 6) for 25–30 minutes.*
- *Remove from the oven and allow to cool, then slice finely.*
- *Add the ingredients of the dressing to a blender and process until smooth, then season to taste.*
- *Place the salad leaves and cucumber on individual plates, top with the beef and drizzle over the dressing.*
- *Garnish with fresh coriander leaves.*

*Carbohydrate content per serving: **5** grams*

Rocket and olive salad

For 2
Handful of rocket leaves
8–10 green olives
1 tbsp freshly squeezed lemon juice
1 tbsp macadamia nut oil
25 grams freshly shaved Parmesan
Freshly ground black pepper

- *Mix the rocket leaves and green olives.*
- *Drizzle the lemon juice and nut oil over the salad, garnish with freshly shaved Parmesan and season with freshly ground black pepper.*

*Carbohydrate content per serving: **1** gram*

Red lettuce salad
The colour tells you that this recipe is high in vitamin A!

For 2   100 grams of mixed red lettuce leaves (radicchio, red oak lettuce, lollo rosso, mignonette)
1 small red pepper, deseeded and sliced thinly
1 red onion, peeled and sliced thinly
4 semi-dried tomatoes with herbs (see page 69)
½ small red chilli, deseeded and chopped finely

* *Mix together the ingredients of the salad and drizzle over the dressing of choice.*

*Carbohydrate content per serving: **11** grams*

Green salad with herbs
Borage is an excellent source of omega-6 essential fatty acid.

For 2   150 grams of mixed green salad leaves (rocket, watercress, dandelion, baby spinach and fresh borage leaves)
2 tsp chopped fresh basil
2 tsp chopped fresh coriander
2 tsp chopped fresh chervil
Pinch of rock salt
Freshly ground black pepper
French vinaigrette (page 206)

* *Mix together the green salad leaves, basil, coriander and chervil, and season to taste.*
* *Drizzle over the vinaigrette.*

*Carbohydrate content per serving: **2** grams*

Crab and herb salad

This is one of the easiest salads to prepare, and one of the most delicious. It really is important to buy good ingredients whenever possible. If you can cook a fresh crab, please do so. We can't, so we always purchase crab ready-cooked! Tinned crab meat is almost as nutritious as fresh, so you can prepare this simple and delicious meal very quickly with just a little forethought when shopping. Remember, the secret of successful dieting is shopping!

For 2
1 large crab, cooked
100 grams mixed green lettuce leaves (frisée, green oak leaf, coral, mizuna and rocket)
1 tbsp chopped fresh basil
1 tbsp chopped fresh chives
1 tsp chopped fresh coriander
Pinch of rock salt
Freshly ground black pepper
Honey and orange vinaigrette (page 207)
Finely chopped spring onions and fresh basil leaves, to garnish

- *Toss the mixed green lettuce leaves, basil, chives and coriander in a large salad bowl and season to taste.*
- *Remove the crab meat from the shell and arrange on the salad, separating the white and dark meat.*
- *Drizzle over the dressing, and garnish with finely chopped spring onions and fresh basil leaves.*

Carbohydrate content per serving: negligible (with 'normal' vinaigrette – page 206); **7** *grams (with honey and orange vinaigrette)*

Chicken and cashew salad
Spinach is rich in vitamins and minerals, but overcooking
prevents the absorption of calcium and iron from the spinach,
so the maximum nutritional value (and best flavour) is ensured
by eating it raw or lightly steamed.

For 2 2 chicken breast fillets, approximately 100–150
grams each
200 grams spinach leaves, washed
1 Lebanese cucumber, sliced lengthways
3 spring onions, chopped into 4–5 cm lengths
1 small Hass avocado, halved, stoned, peeled and
thinly sliced
1 tbsp chopped fresh basil
50 grams raw cashew nuts
25 grams pine nuts
Freshly ground black pepper
Lemon and coriander vinaigrette (page 208)

- *Place the chicken fillets in a shallow oven-safe dish
and dot with butter.*
- *Cover with perforated aluminium foil and cook in the
centre of a pre-heated oven at 180°C (gas mark 4)
for 40–45 minutes.*
- *Remove with a perforated spoon and set aside to
cool. When cool, slice on the diagonal into 2–3 cm
slices.*
- *Arrange the spinach on the plates. Toss the
cucumber, spring onions, avocado and basil with the
nuts, and spoon onto the spinach.*
- *Place the chicken on the salad and drizzle over the
dressing.*

*Carbohydrate content per serving: **10** grams*

Asparagus and parma ham salad

Vitamin B_1 from Parma ham, vitamin D from Parmesan cheese and vitamin A from asparagus are only some of the essential nutrients provided by this delicious recipe.

For 2   150 grams asparagus, trimmed
75 grams rocket
3 slices Parma ham, finely sliced
1 tbsp chopped fresh chives
30 grams freshly shaved Parmesan cheese
Pinch of rock salt
Freshly ground black pepper
Pine nuts, to garnish
Lemon and coriander vinaigrette (page 208)

- *Lightly steam the asparagus until tender but still firm.*
- *Mix together the asparagus, rocket, Parma ham, chives and Parmesan, and season to taste.*
- *Drizzle over lemon and coriander vinaigrette, and garnish with pine nuts.*

Carbohydrate content per serving: 2 grams

Vegetable salad

Oriental vinaigrette adds zest to this colourful and nutritious salad.

For 2   75 grams mangetout
50 grams French beans
1 small yellow pepper, deseeded and thinly sliced
1 small red pepper, deseeded and thinly sliced
3 spring onions, chopped into 4–5 cm lengths on the
    diagonal
3 baby yellow squash, quartered vertically
Freshly ground black pepper
Oriental vinaigrette (page 207)
Lime zest and fresh basil leaves, to garnish

- *Lightly steam the vegetables, then pour over the dressing.*
- *Garnish with lime zest and fresh basil leaves.*

Carbohydrate content per serving: 8 grams

Crispy green salad

For 2   100 grams mixed crispy lettuce leaves (cos, curly
endive, coral, green oak leaf and mizuna)
1 medium Lebanese cucumber, sliced lengthways
1 celery stick, chopped on the diagonal
1 small green pepper, deseeded and thinly sliced
1 small ripe Hass avocado, halved, stoned and diced
Fresh basil leaves, to garnish

Dressing
4 tbsp extra-virgin olive oil
1 tbsp white wine vinegar
Freshly ground black pepper
Pinch of sugar
1 tsp Dijon mustard

- *Place the dressing ingredients in a screw-top jar and mix well.*
- *Toss the green salad in a large salad bowl and pour the dressing over. Garnish with fresh basil.*

Carbohydrate content per serving: 6 grams

Char-grilled pepper salad with herb mayonnaise

For 2   1 medium red pepper, deseeded and quartered
         1 medium green pepper, deseeded and quartered
         1 medium yellow pepper, deseeded and quartered
         1 red onion, peeled and quartered
         1 fennel bulb, peeled and quartered
         2 tbsp extra-virgin olive oil
         Handful of red oak leaf lettuce leaves
         Fresh coriander leaves, to garnish

Herb mayonnaise

         1 tbsp chopped fresh thyme
         1 tbsp chopped fresh parsley
         1 tsp chopped fresh coriander
         100 ml mayonnaise (page 210)

- *Mix the chopped fresh parsley and thyme into the mayonnaise.*
- *Place the peppers (skin uppermost), onion and fennel bulb in a single layer on a grill tray.*
- *Brush with olive oil and cook under a pre-heated grill for about 5 minutes, or until the skin of the peppers blisters.*
- *Peel the peppers and remove the outer skin of the onion and fennel, then slice them into thin strips and allow to cool.*
- *Arrange the vegetables on a bed of red oak leaf lettuce leaves in a shallow dish, top with the herb mayonnaise and garnish with fresh coriander leaves.*

*Carbohydrate content per serving: **11** grams*

Tomatoes and mozzarella with mango dressing

For 2   2 large vine-ripened tomatoes, thickly sliced
100 grams of mozzarella, sliced
Slices of mango and lime zest, to garnish

Dressing

4 tbsp extra-virgin olive oil
1 tbsp white wine vinegar
2 slices fresh mango, puréed
½ tsp sesame seeds
Pinch of rock salt
Freshly ground black pepper

- *Place the dressing ingredients in a screw-top jar and shake well.*
- *Place slices of tomato and mozzarella alternately around the circumference of a plate and drizzle over the dressing.*
- *Garnish with slices of mango and lime zest.*

Carbohydrate content per serving: 5 grams

Tomato, ginger and orange salad

For 2   4 large vine-ripened tomatoes, cubed
1 large sweet orange, peeled
1 tbsp extra-virgin olive oil
2 tsp ginger wine
Freshly ground black pepper
Fresh basil leaves, to garnish

- *Divide the orange into segments, remove all the centre pith and pips, and chop into small 2–3 cm segments.*
- *Add the tomato segments, drizzle over 1 tbsp of virgin olive oil and 2 tsp of ginger wine, and mix thoroughly.*
- *Chill for at least 30 minutes, season with freshly ground black pepper and garnish with fresh basil leaves.*

*Carbohydrate content per serving: **11** grams*

Chicken breast with chilli sauce

If you decide to cook the chicken breast rather than purchase ready-cooked, remember to cook the chicken the previous evening. Realistically, there will not be time in the morning to cook chicken, so with a little (and we mean very little) preparation the previous evening, you can enjoy a delicious (and relatively inexpensive) lunch-on-the-run.

For 1   1 chicken breast
25 grams unsalted butter, cubed
½ Lebanese cucumber, cubed
4 cherry tomatoes on the vine, halved
2 tsp chilli sauce
30 grams (approximately) rocket and watercress leaves
Freshly ground black pepper

- *Place the chicken breast in an oven-safe dish and dot with cubes of butter.*
- *Cover with pierced aluminium foil and cook in the centre of a pre-heated oven at 180°C (gas mark 4) for 35–40 minutes, then set aside to cool.*
  (Or use a purchased ready-cooked chicken breast.)
- *Slice the cooked chicken breast and mix with the cucumber, tomatoes and chilli sauce in a medium bowl.*
- *Lay a bed of rocket and watercress leaves in the base of the lunchbox and top with the chilli chicken mixture.*
- *Season to taste with freshly ground black pepper.*

*Carbohydrate content per serving: **4 grams***

Roast ham with Leerdammer cheese and mustard

For 1   30 grams (approximately) red lettuce salad leaves
(radiccio, red oak lettuce, lollo rosso)
Drizzle of French vinaigrette (page 206)
2–3 slices thick honey-roast ham (from the deli or
supermarket)
1 slice Leerdammer cheese (pre-sliced from
supermarket)
1 tsp wholegrain mustard
Freshly ground black pepper

- *Lay a bed of red lettuce salad in the lunchbox.*
- *Drizzle over a little French vinaigrette. This can be easily home-made and stored for later use, or use commercial.*
- *Top with the honey-roast ham and Leerdammer cheese, with 1 tsp of delicious wholegrain mustard.*
- *Season to taste with freshly ground black pepper.*

Carbohydrate content per serving: 1 gram

Tuna mayonnaise with basil and coriander

For 1   200 gram tin tuna (in brine), drained and flaked
1 tbsp mayonnaise (page 210)
2 tsp chopped fresh basil
2 tsp chopped fresh coriander
1 spring onion, finely chopped
30 grams (approximately) fresh watercress
Freshly ground black pepper

- *Mix together the tuna, mayonnaise, basil, coriander and spring onion in a medium bowl.*
- *Lay a bed of watercress in the base of the lunchbox and top with the tuna mixture.*
- *Season to taste with freshly ground black pepper.*

Carbohydrate content per serving: 1 gram

Salmon with crème fraîche

For 1   1 medium salmon fillet, approximately 125–150 grams
        30 grams unsalted butter, cubed
        ¼ Lebanese cucumber, diced
        1 tsp chopped fresh chives
        75 ml crème fraîche
        30 grams (approximately) wild rocket leaves
        Drizzle of French vinaigrette (page 206)
        2 small plum tomatoes on the vine, halved
        Freshly ground black pepper

- *Place the salmon fillet in a shallow oven-safe dish, dot with butter, cover with pierced aluminium foil and cook in the centre of a pre-heated oven at 180°C (gas mark 4) for 12–15 minutes.*

Or

- *Place the salmon fillet in a microwave-safe dish, pour over a tablespoon of water, cover and cook on 'high' for 2½ minutes, then allow to stand for a further minute.*

At the same time
- *Mix together the cucumber, chives and crème fraîche in a small bowl.*
- *Lay a bed of wild rocket leaves in the base of the lunchbox and drizzle over some French vinaigrette.*
- *Place the salmon fillet on the rocket.*
- *Arrange the tomatoes around the salmon and spoon the cucumber crème fraîche onto the salmon.*
- *Season to taste with freshly ground black pepper.*

*Carbohydrate content per serving: **4** grams*

Tiger prawns with chilli and coriander vinaigrette
This is so simple to prepare, provided you plan to have the
ingredients available, and so delicious. We would strongly
advise you to make your own vinaigrette rather than buy a
commercial variety. It takes moments to make, is much less
expensive and can be adapted in many different ways. Of
course, a commercial vinaigrette is just as effective – but
always remember to check the carbohydrate content as it can
vary from virtually zero to unacceptable levels! The vinaigrettes
to avoid are the 'low-fat' variety as they are usually higher in
carbohydrate content.

For 1   1 tsp chopped fresh coriander
          ¼ green chilli, deseeded and finely diced
          2 tbsp French vinaigrette, home-made (page 206) or
             commercial
          8 pre-cooked tiger prawns, shelled
          1 small yellow pepper, deseeded and diced
          30 grams (approximately) watercress and rocket
             salad leaves
          Freshly ground black pepper

- *Mix together the coriander, chilli and vinaigrette in a
  medium bowl.*
- *Stir in the tiger prawns and diced yellow pepper, and
  marinate for at least 20 minutes (preferably
  overnight). If you don't have any time in the morning
  omit the marinating period.*
- *Place the watercress and rocket leaves in the base of
  the lunchbox and top up with the tiger prawns in chilli
  and coriander vinaigrette.*
- *Season to taste with freshly ground black pepper.*

*Carbohydrate content per serving: **3** grams*

Chicken and wild rocket salad

For 2   2 chicken breasts, approximately 125–150 grams
        each
        30 grams unsalted butter
        6 cherry vine tomatoes, halved
        1 medium Hass avocado, peeled, stone removed and
        chopped
        1 tbsp chopped fresh coriander
        1 tbsp chopped fresh chives
        75 grams wild rocket leaves
        Drizzle of French vinaigrette (page 206)
        Freshly ground black pepper

- *Place the chicken breasts in an oven-safe dish and dot with butter.*
- *Cover with pierced aluminium foil and cook in the centre of a pre-heated oven at 180°C (gas mark 4) for 35–40 minutes, then set aside to cool.*
  (Or use two chicken breasts which have been purchased ready-cooked.)
- *Chop the chicken breast into cubes.*
- *Mix together the chicken breast, tomatoes, avocado, coriander, chives and wild rocket in a large salad bowl, drizzle over some French vinaigrette and season to taste with freshly ground black pepper.*
- *Serve immediately.*

Carbohydrate content per serving: 6 grams

Grilled red mullet and avocado salad

For 2   4 medium red mullet, cleaned
        Extra-virgin olive oil
        1 medium Hass avocado, peeled, chopped and stone
        removed
        8 cherry tomatoes, halved
        1 tbsp chopped fresh flat-leaf parsley
        50 grams wild rocket
        Freshly ground black pepper
        Lemon vinaigrette (page 209)

- *Brush the red mullet with extra-virgin olive oil, then place under a medium grill for 8 minutes, turning once.*
- *Toss the avocado, tomatoes, parsley and rocket, and season to taste with freshly ground black pepper.*
- *Drizzle over a little lemon vinaigrette.*
- *Serve the mullet with the salad.*

Carbohydrate content per serving: 6 grams

Fennel and herb salad

For 2   1 bulb Florence fennel, washed and chopped
1 spring onion, chopped on the diagonal into 2–3 cm
   lengths
50 grams mangetout, topped and tailed
75 grams fresh watercress
1 tbsp chopped fresh basil
1 tbsp chopped fresh chives
Freshly ground black pepper
French vinaigrette (page 206)

- *Toss the ingredients of the salad, season to taste with freshly ground black pepper and drizzle over a little vinaigrette.*
- *Serve immediately.*

Carbohydrate content per serving: 8 grams

Salmon and basil pâté

The king of herbs with the king of fish. The term 'basil' is derived from the Greek word for 'king', which is most appropriate for such a nutritious and versatile herb. Apart from its undoubted gastronomic uses, basil has also been used as a mild tranquilliser for centuries. You can use fresh or tinned salmon. The tinned variety has similar nutritional qualities as fresh salmon; it still has excellent flavour, but not quite as good as its fresh counterpart.

For 2
400 grams salmon fillet (or 440 gram tin of red salmon, drained and bones removed)
100 ml full-cream milk
25 grams butter
2 shallots, peeled and finely chopped
1 garlic clove, peeled and finely chopped
1 tbsp freshly squeezed lemon juice
2 tbsp Chardonnay
1 tbsp chopped fresh basil
1 tsp chopped fresh coriander
2 tbsp freshly grated breadcrumbs (one small slice of toasted bread – wholemeal or white)
2 egg whites
50 grams melted butter
Freshly ground black pepper
Sprigs of fresh coriander, to garnish

- *Place the salmon fillet in a baking dish and pour the milk around the salmon.*
- *Cover with pierced aluminium foil and cook in the centre of a preheated oven at 180°C (gas mark 4) for about 20 minutes.*
- *Remove from the oven and set aside to cool.*

Or instead you could
- Replace the above with 440 grams of tinned red salmon, drained and bones removed.

Then
- Heat 25 grams of butter in a small saucepan and sauté the shallots and garlic for 2–3 minutes.
- Flake the salmon in a medium mixing bowl, add the shallots, garlic, lemon juice, Chardonnay, basil, coriander, breadcrumbs, egg whites and melted butter.
- Season to taste and mix thoroughly.
- Line a loaf tin with aluminium foil and press the pâté mixture firmly in the base of the tin.
- Close the foil parcel loosely, and cook in the centre of a preheated oven at 180°C (gas mark 4) for 40–45 minutes.
- Remove and set aside to cool before serving.

*Carbohydrate content per serving: **16** grams*

Smoked trout pâté

Fats in your diet don't necessarily make you fat! In fact, they only cause weight gain when combined with carbohydrates, so include some of the 'good' pure fats (like cheese) in your diet for health: fats slow the digestive process and satisfy hunger, actually encouraging you to eat less! Cheese and cream (in moderation) are definitely beneficial, not harmful.

Horseradish is a rich source of vitamin C and a gastric stimulant. In this recipe, it blends perfectly with the powerful flavour of smoked trout.

For 2
1 smoked trout, flaked and boned
150 grams Philadelphia cheese
1 tbsp horseradish sauce (page 215)
2 tbsp single cream
1 tbsp chopped fresh basil
2 tsp chopped fresh coriander
Pinch of rock salt
Freshly ground black pepper
Pinch of paprika and fresh basil leaves, to garnish

- *Mix together the smoked trout, cheese, horseradish sauce, cream, basil and coriander, then season to taste.*
- *Blend until smooth and chill for 3–4 hours in the fridge.*
- *Just before serving, garnish with fresh basil leaves and paprika.*

Carbohydrate content per serving: 4 grams

Taramasalata

Try to be adventurous – particularly with fish. Seafood has a natural variety of different tastes and textures. Providing they are not overcooked (and ruined), you can gently merge different tastes with the natural saltiness of the sea. Smoked cod roe is deliciously complemented, both nutritionally and gastronomically, by chives and green salad.

For 2
1 thin slice white bread, crust removed
2 tbsp full-cream milk
150 grams smoked cod roe, skin removed
½ garlic clove, peeled and finely chopped
½ small brown onion, peeled and finely grated
3 tbsp extra-virgin olive oil
1 tbsp freshly squeezed lemon juice
Freshly ground black pepper
Chopped fresh chives, to garnish
Crispy green salad (page 79)

- *Soak the bread in the milk, drain through a sieve and finely chop.*
- *Stir in the cod roe, onion and garlic, and mix in the virgin olive oil gradually.*
- *Add the lemon juice and season to taste with freshly ground black pepper (salt will probably not be necessary as cod roe is naturally salty).*
- *Blend until smooth and chill in the fridge for 3–4 hours before serving.*
- *Just before serving, garnish with chopped fresh chives and serve with crispy green salad.*

*Carbohydrate content per serving: **11** grams (including salad)*

Spicy chicken drumsticks

For 2
6 chicken drumsticks, skin on, scored diagonally on each side
2 tbsp extra-virgin olive oil
Julienne strips of green chilli, to garnish

Marinade
2 tbsp light soy sauce
2 tbsp sweet sherry
1 garlic clove, peeled and finely chopped
2 slices of fresh ginger root, peeled and finely chopped
1 tsp sesame oil

- *Mix the soy sauce, sherry, garlic, ginger and sesame oil in a medium bowl, add the drumsticks and marinate for 3–4 hours.*
- *Brush the drumsticks with extra-virgin olive oil, and barbecue (or grill) for about 10–12 minutes, turning regularly and basting with the marinade.*

*Carbohydrate content per serving: **3** grams*

Savoury crêpes

Savoury crêpes are perfect for light lunch, supper or even breakfast! As each crêpe contains only 5–6 grams of carbohydrate (or about one-third of the amount of carbohydrate in a single slice of bread) you can enjoy crêpes in moderation as the crêpe itself is only a transport medium for the filling, and you can be as adventurous as you want in designer, quickly prepared, low-carb fillings. This recipe can be made by hand or using a blender.

For 2
50 grams plain flour
Pinch of salt
1 large free-range egg, beaten
150 ml full-cream milk
1 tbsp melted butter

- *Sieve the flour and salt into a medium bowl.*
- *Add ½ of the beaten egg mixture, whisking constantly.*
- *Gradually blend in the milk, drawing the mixture to the centre of the bowl until you achieve an even consistency.*
- *Allow to stand for at least ½ hour before making the crêpes.*
- *Just before cooking, stir the melted butter into the mixture.*

Traditional method

- *Add a level tablespoon of butter to a small non-stick frying pan, melt the butter over medium heat and evenly coat the pan.*
- *Add 2 tablespoons of the mixture to the pan, then tip the pan to evenly coat the base of the pan. Cook for about 20–30 seconds and remove with a palette knife.*

Crêpe-maker

- *Pour the mixture into a wide shallow dish.*
- *Turn on the crêpe-maker. When hot, dip the crêpe-maker horizonally onto the mixture to lightly coat and allow the crêpe to cook. When the edge of the crêpe is lightly browned, remove with a palette knife and repeat the process.*

Savoury crêpes can either be rolled around the selected filling, folded in half over the filling or folded into triangles and topped with the savoury filling.

. . . .

Prawn mayonnaise crêpes

For 2   6 crêpes (as above)
100 grams pre-cooked prawns
1 tbsp mayonnaise (page 210)
½ tbsp chopped fresh coriander
½ tbsp chopped fresh chives
Pinch of cayenne pepper

- *Prepare the crêpes.*

At the same time

- *Mix together the prawns, mayonnaise, coriander and chives.*
- *Stir in a pinch of cayenne pepper.*
- *Spoon the mixture evenly over the crêpes, then fold the crêpes in half and serve immediately.*

Carbohydrate content per serving (3 crêpes): **15 grams**

Spinach and Emmental crêpes

For 2   6 crêpes (as above)
15 grams unsalted butter
15 grams plain flour
150 ml full-cream milk
100 grams Emmental cheese, grated
75 grams spinach leaves
1 tbsp chopped fresh flat-leaf parsley
Freshly ground black pepper

- *Prepare the crêpes.*
- *Melt the butter in a medium saucepan, remove from the heat and stir in the flour.*
- *Return to a low heat and gradually blend in the milk.*
- *When the sauce begins to thicken, stir in the grated Emmental cheese.*
- *Season to taste.*

At the same time
- *Lightly steam (or microwave) the spinach for 3–4 minutes.*
- *Chop the spinach leaves and mix with the chopped parsley.*

- *Mix the spinach and parsley into the cheese sauce. Spoon the mixture evenly over the crêpes, then fold the crêpes in half.*
- *Serve immediately.*

*Carbohydrate content per serving (3 crêpes): **26** grams*

Haddock with herbs

Buy fresh fish when you can (either from the fishmonger or supermarket) and freeze it for later use, or buy frozen fish fillets (without batter, breadcrumbs or dressing).

For 2
2 medium haddock fillets
2 shallots, peeled and finely chopped
1 tbsp chopped fresh flat-leaf parsley
1 tbsp chopped fresh coriander
2 slices fresh root ginger, peeled and finely chopped
100 ml dry white wine
Freshly ground black pepper
Sprigs of fresh dill, to garnish

- *Place the haddock fillets in an oven-safe dish and top with the shallots, parsley, coriander and ginger.*
- *Pour the wine over the fish, cover with pierced aluminium foil and cook in the centre of a pre-heated oven at 180°C (gas mark 4) for 15–18 minutes.*
- *Season to taste and serve immediately, garnished with sprigs of fresh dill.*

Quick method

- *Place the haddock fillets in a microwave-safe dish and top with the shallots, parsley, coriander and ginger.*
- *Pour 2 tbsp wine over the fish, cover with the appropriate cover for the container (not aluminium foil!) and cook in the centre of a microwave oven (850W) for 2½ minutes. Increase the time by a third (to about 3 minutes) for a 650–750W oven.*
- *Season to taste and serve immediately, garnished with sprigs of fresh dill.*

Carbohydrate content per serving: 2 grams

Penne rigate with mixed veg

For 2   25 grams mangetout
25 grams broccoli florets
1 small red pepper, deseeded and finely sliced
40 grams wholemeal penne rigate
75 ml double cream
1 tbsp freshly chopped basil
1 tbsp freshly grated Parmesan cheese
Freshly ground black pepper

- *Lightly steam the mangetout, broccoli florets and red pepper for 4–5 minutes (or microwave on 'high' for 2–3 minutes).*

At the same time
- *Cook the penne rigate.*
- *Mix together the double cream and basil.*
- *Stir the mangetout, broccoli and red pepper into the penne rigate, stir in the cream and Parmesan cheese, and season to taste with freshly ground black pepper.*

*Carbohydrate content per serving: **20** grams*

Avocado and smoked salmon with dill mayonnaise
Quick and simple – but highly nutritious and delicious!

For 2   Medium Hass avocado, peeled, stone removed and
             sliced
          75 grams smoked salmon, sliced into thin strips
          1 tbsp freshly squeezed lime juice
          Freshly ground black pepper

Dill mayonnaise
          2 tbsp mayonnaise – commercial, or home-made
             (page 210)
          ½ tbsp finely chopped fresh dill

*   *Divide avocado slices evenly between two plates and
    place in the centre.*
*   *Lay several strips of smoked salmon on the avocado.*
*   *Drizzle the lime juice over the salmon.*

At the same time
*   *Mix together the mayonnaise and dill.*
*   *Spoon the dill mayonnaise on to the salmon and
    season to taste with freshly ground black pepper.*

*Carbohydrate content per serving: **3** grams*

Chapter **8** Quick-and-easy dinner

Delicious low-GI dinners can be quick-and-easy; the secret is to plan ahead. Make sure you have all of the basics in your store-cupboard (see page 23) and plan your meals for the week when you are shopping to make sure you have all the essentials for dinner every day in advance.

Poultry

Tarragon chicken

For 2   250–300 grams skinless chicken breast
         75 ml mayonnaise (page 210, or buy ready-made)
         1 tbsp chopped fresh tarragon
         Pinch of rock salt
         Freshly ground black pepper
         Sprigs of fresh tarragon, to garnish

• *Bake the chicken as described on page 76 allow to cool, then slice thinly.*
• *Stir the chopped tarragon into the mayonnaise and season to taste.*
• *Arrange the chicken slices on the plate and top with the tarragon mayonnaise.*
• *Serve garnished with sprigs of fresh tarragon.*

Carbohydrate content per serving: negligible

Chicken tikka
A delicious dish, not too spicy, which combines the natural proteins, vitamins and minerals of the chicken with the vitamins and antioxidants of the herbs.

For 2   300 grams skinless chicken breast, cubed

Marinade
½ tsp chilli powder
1 garlic clove, peeled and finely chopped
2 slices fresh ginger root, peeled and finely chopped
½ tsp ground turmeric
½ tsp ground cumin
1 shallot, peeled and grated
Pinch of rock salt
Freshly ground black pepper
2 tsp fresh lemon juice
100 ml natural yoghurt
2 tsp fresh coriander, finely chopped

- *Mix together the chilli powder, garlic, ginger, turmeric, cumin, shallot, salt, pepper, lemon juice, natural yoghurt and coriander in a medium bowl, and stir in the chicken. Cover and leave to marinate in the fridge for at least 3–4 hours – or preferably overnight.*
- *Grill the marinated chicken under medium heat for about 20 minutes, turning regularly.*
- *Serve with a crispy green salad (see page 79) and lime wedges.*

*Carbohydrate content per serving: **11** grams*

Lemon chicken with cashew nuts

For 2   3 tbsp extra-virgin olive oil
250 grams skinless chicken breast, thinly sliced
50 grams raw cashew nuts
Lemon wedges
Lemon zest to garnish
75 grams mangetout
75 grams broccoli florets

Sauce   1 tsp cornflour
2 tbsp water
Juice of a freshly squeezed lemon
1 tbsp light soy sauce
2 tbsp sweet sherry

- *Prepare the cornflour mixture by adding the cornflour to 2 tbsp of water, stirring to ensure an even consistency.*
- *Heat the olive oil in the wok, then stir-fry the chicken breast strips on medium heat for about 3–4 minutes, stirring frequently.*
- *Remove the chicken to a casserole dish, mix with the cashew nuts, cover and place in a warm oven. Drain the wok and wipe clean.*
- *Mix together the lemon juice, soy sauce and sherry in a bowl, and stir in the cornflour paste, mixing to an even consistency.*
- *Transfer to the wok and heat to a gentle simmer, stirring constantly for about 1–2 minutes, until the sauce thickens.*
- *Return the chicken and cashew nuts to the wok and simmer for 2–3 minutes.*
- *Lightly steam the mangetout and broccoli florets. Garnish the chicken with lemon zest and serve with the vegetables.*

*Carbohydrate content per serving: **15** grams*

Chicken with tomato and basil sauce

For 2
2 skinless chicken breasts (about 150 grams each)
25 grams butter, cubed
3 tbsp extra-virgin olive oil
1 medium onion, peeled and chopped
1 garlic clove, peeled and finely chopped
400 gram tin of plum tomatoes
1 tbsp tomato purée
50 ml dry white wine
75 ml chicken stock
75 grams button mushrooms, wiped and halved
1 tbsp chopped fresh basil
Pinch of rock salt
Freshly ground black pepper
Fresh basil leaves, to garnish
100 grams broccoli florets
100 grams carrots, julienned

- *Place the chicken breasts in the base of a shallow casserole dish, arrange the cubes of butter on the chicken, then cover with pierced aluminium foil and cook in centre of a preheated oven at 180°C (gas mark 4) for 35–40 minutes.*
- *Remove the fillets with a perforated spoon and allow to cool, then chop into large cubes.*
- *Heat the olive oil in a large frying pan and sauté the onion and garlic for 1–2 minutes.*
- *Add the tomatoes, tomato purée, white wine, stock and mushrooms, then simmer for 6–8 minutes.*
- *Stir in the chopped basil and chicken, season to taste and simmer for a further 15 minutes.*
- *Lightly steam the broccoli and carrots. Garnish the chicken with fresh basil leaves and serve.*

Carbohydrate content per serving: 17 grams

Chicken with prosciutto

The cheese in this recipe can be varied according to taste –
it is equally delicious with Edam, Emmental, Gruyère or
Jarlsberg. We consider strong cheeses (such as some
Cheddars and Stilton) to be too overpowering for this
combination.

For 2
2 skinless chicken breast fillets (about 150 grams
each)
2 tbsp plain flour, seasoned
2 tbsp extra-virgin olive oil
1 tbsp fresh basil, finely chopped
4 large slices of prosciutto
30 grams freshly grated Parmesan cheese
Freshly ground black pepper
1 tsp chopped fresh chives, to garnish
1 tsp chopped fresh coriander, to garnish

- *Using a sharp knife, slice each chicken breast
  lengthways into two thin, flat halves. Season the flour
  with salt and black pepper and lightly coat the
  chicken breasts with it.*
- *Heat the olive oil in a frying pan, add the chicken
  fillets and chopped basil, and cook over a moderate
  heat for 8–10 minutes, turning twice, until evenly
  cooked on both sides.*
- *Remove the chicken to a grill-pan, place a slice of
  prosciutto on each fillet and sprinkle grated
  Parmesan cheese on the prosciutto. Season with
  freshly ground black pepper and place under a
  preheated grill until the cheese has just melted.*
- *Serve garnished with fresh chives and coriander.*

*Carbohydrate content per serving: **12** grams*

Mozzarella chicken
This delicious meal is ideal for a light lunch or supper. And incredibly healthy: protein from chicken and mozzarella, lycopene and vitamin A from tomato, antioxidants par excellence from the coriander and chives ... the list is endless.

For 2
2 skinless chicken breast fillets, approximately
   100–125 grams each
25 grams butter, cubed
1 large vine-ripened tomato, thickly sliced
1 tbsp chopped fresh chives
2 tsp chopped fresh coriander
4–6 thin slices of mozzarella cheese
Freshly ground black pepper
75 grams wild rocket
Passata vinaigrette (page 206)
Fresh coriander leaves, to garnish

- *Flatten the chicken fillets and place in a medium baking dish. Dot with cubes of butter, cover with pierced aluminium foil and cook in the centre of a preheated oven at 180°C (gas mark 4) for 35–40 minutes.*
- *Remove the chicken fillets with a perforated spoon and transfer them to a grill tray.*
- *Top with slices of tomato, sprinkle over the herbs and add a final layer of thin slices of mozzarella.*
- *Grill under a hot grill (approximately 8–10 cm from the grill) until the cheese has melted.*
- *Serve on a bed of wild rocket, drizzle over a little passata vinaigrette and garnish with fresh coriander leaves.*

*Carbohydrate content per serving: **4** grams*

Spicy turkey kebabs

For some unknown reason, roast turkey seems to be inextricably linked with Yuletide – and no other time of year. In fact, nothing could be further from the truth. Turkey can now be bought in the same way as chicken, either as whole breast fillets (or ready sliced breast) or drumsticks. As with all pure foods, turkey has a unique taste and texture, and the ability to absorb appropriate flavours. In this recipe, the delicate aroma of the spices blends with the tangy lemon, and is tempered by the cooling influence of the yoghurt.

For 2   2 skinless turkey breast fillets (approximately
            150 grams each), cubed
          Crispy green salad (page 79)

Marinade
          2 tsp ground cumin
          1 tsp ground coriander
          2 tsp garam masala
          ½ tsp ground ginger
          1 garlic clove, peeled and grated
          1 tbsp freshly squeezed lemon juice
          125 ml natural yoghurt

- *Grate the garlic with a ginger- or garlic-grater.*
- *Prepare the marinade and marinate the turkey for 4–6 hours in the fridge.*
- *Remember to soak the wooden skewers during this period, or they will burn when you grill later.*
- *Thread the skewers with the marinated turkey cubes and cook under a medium grill, no closer than 8 cm from the grill, for about 8–10 minutes, turning frequently.*

- *Serve immediately with a crispy green salad.*

*Carbohydrate content per serving: **5** grams (including salad)*

. . . .

Basil pesto turkey with char-grilled vegetables and sesame seeds

This is a delicious light lunch, full of healthy nutrition. Pine nuts are an excellent source of vitamin B_1 and vitamin E with the dietary advantage of a relatively low carbohydrate content.

For 2   Basil pesto sauce (page 209)
200 grams turkey breast fillet, sliced
Char-grilled vegetables with sesame seeds
   (page 172)
Fresh oregano leaves, to garnish

- *Prepare the pesto sauce.*
- *Coat the slices of turkey breast with pesto sauce and marinate for 3–4 hours.*
- *Place on a grill tray under a medium grill, approximately 8 cm from the heat, and grill for 8–10 minutes, turning once.*

At the same time
- *Char-grill the vegetables.*
- *Serve the basil pesto turkey with char-grilled vegetables, garnished with fresh oregano leaves.*

*Carbohydrate content per serving: **14** grams (only **2** grams without vegetables)*

Chilli mayonnaise turkey with mangetout

This dish is just as delicious with normal mayonnaise (page 210) or creamy curry mayonnaise (page 211); it simply depends on individual taste. The carbohydrate content is the same for all.

For 2   4 tbsp extra-virgin olive oil
    350 grams turkey breast fillet, thinly sliced
    50 ml chilli mayonnaise (page 216)
    50 grams French beans
    100 grams mangetout
    3 spring onions, finely chopped
    1 garlic clove, peeled and finely chopped
    2 slices of fresh ginger root, peeled and finely chopped
    Pinch of rock salt
    Freshly ground black pepper

- *Prepare the mayonnaise according to the recipe you prefer.*
- *Heat 2 tbsp of extra-virgin olive oil in a wok and stir-fry the turkey breast for 4–5 minutes.*
- *Remove from the wok, pat dry and allow to cool.*
- *Mix the turkey breast with the mayonnaise.*
- *Heat the remaining 2 tbsp of virgin olive oil in the wok and stir-fry the French beans for 3–4 minutes.*
- *Add the mangetout, spring onions, garlic and ginger.*
- *Season to taste and stir-fry for 3–4 minutes.*
- *Serve immediately with the turkey and mayonnaise.*

*Carbohydrate content per serving: **4 grams***

Coconut chicken with pine nuts

Ready in minutes, this tastes delicious and is high in healthy antioxidants.

For 2
2 skinless chicken breasts, about 150 grams each, sliced
1 tbsp freshly squeezed lemon juice
2 tbsp extra-virgin olive oil
1 garlic clove, peeled and finely chopped
3 spring onions, finely chopped
1 yellow pepper, deseeded and finely sliced
30 grams pine nuts, crushed
1 tbsp chopped fresh basil
1 tbsp chopped fresh flat-leaf parsley
2 plum tomatoes, chopped
50 ml coconut milk
2–3 drops Tabasco sauce (optional)
Pinch of rock salt
Freshly ground black pepper
Chopped fresh chives, to garnish

- *Drizzle the lemon juice over the chicken.*
- *Heat the olive oil in a wok and brown the chicken.*
- *Stir in the garlic, spring onions, pepper and pine nuts, and stir-fry over medium heat for 2–3 minutes.*
- *Add the basil, parsley, tomatoes, coconut milk, and Tabasco sauce if desired, and season to taste.*
- *Simmer gently for 10 minutes.*
- *Serve immediately, garnished with chopped fresh chives.*

Carbohydrate content per serving: **9** *grams*

Chicken satay with lime

Freshly ground black pepper is included in many recipes, not just for taste, but also because ground black pepper contains a high concentration of the mineral chromium, which we need for the functioning of our pancreas and which is important in the prevention of diabetes.

For 2
250 grams chicken breast fillets, skinned and cubed
200 grams fresh spinach leaves
1 lime, quartered
Freshly ground black pepper

Satay sauce

2 shallots, peeled and diced
1 garlic clove, peeled and crushed
2 tsp medium curry powder
2 tbsp peanut butter
1 tbsp liquid honey
3 tbsp soy sauce

- *Mix together the ingredients for the marinade and marinate the chicken for 3–4 hours.*
- *Soak two wooden skewers in cold water for 5–10 minutes before cooking.*
- *Thread the chicken cubes onto the wooden skewers.*
- *Grill under a hot grill, 8–10 cm from the flame, or barbecue, for 8–10 minutes, turning regularly.*

At the same time

- *Lightly steam the spinach for 4–5 minutes or microwave the spinach for 3–4 minutes.*
- *Serve the chicken satay kebabs on a bed of spinach, drizzle over some freshly squeezed lime juice and season to taste.*

*Carbohydrate content per serving: **10 grams***

Honey and ginger chicken

The flavour of chicken blends perfectly with the sweetness of the honey and the spicy ginger. And both peppers and chilli are members of the capsicum family, which is well-known to be an excellent source of the antioxidant vitamins A and C. Once again, it simply proves that healthy food tastes delicious, if prepared correctly.

For 2
- 2 chicken breast fillets, sliced into thin strips
- 3 tbsp extra-virgin olive oil
- 1 red onion, peeled and sliced vertically into wedges
- 1 medium yellow pepper, deseeded and chopped into large cubes
- 1 medium red pepper, deseeded and chopped into large cubes
- 1 tbsp chopped fresh basil
- Freshly ground black pepper
- Fresh basil leaves, to garnish

Marinade
- 2 slices fresh ginger root, peeled and finely chopped
- 1 green chilli, deseeded and finely chopped
- 1 garlic clove, peeled and finely chopped
- 2 tbsp light soy sauce
- 2 tbsp sweet sherry
- 1 tbsp clear honey
- Juice of half a lemon, freshly squeezed

- *Mix together the ingredients of the marinade, and marinate the chicken strips for 3–4 hours.*
- *Heat 2 tbsp of extra-virgin olive oil in the wok, and stir-fry the onion and peppers for 2–3 minutes.*

- *Remove from the wok with a perforated spoon and set aside.*
- *Heat the remaining olive oil in the wok and stir-fry the chicken strips for 2–3 minutes.*
- *Add the remaining marinade and stir-fry for another minute.*
- *Return the vegetables to the wok, add the basil and season to taste.*
- *Stir-fry for 1 final minute before serving, garnished with fresh basil leaves.*

*Carbohydrate content per serving: **19** grams*

Thai chicken with lemongrass and ginger
Ginger has been recognised for its medicinal properties since
ancient times. It is said to improve circulation and prevent
blood coagulation, as well as improve digestion.

For 2
250 grams chicken breast fillets
50 grams butter, cubed
3 tbsp extra-virgin olive oil
1 medium red onion, peeled and sliced
1 medium garlic clove, peeled and finely sliced
2 stalks lemongrass, husk removed and finely chopped
1 green chilli, deseeded and finely chopped (optional)
3 slices fresh ginger root, peeled and finely chopped
1 tbsp tamarind paste
1 medium red pepper, deseeded and sliced
1 medium green pepper, deseeded and sliced
100 grams mangetout
400 ml coconut milk
Freshly ground black pepper

- *Place the chicken breast fillets in a shallow baking
  dish, dot with butter cubes and cover with pierced
  aluminium foil.*
- *Cook in the centre of a preheated oven at 180°C
  (gas mark 4) for 35–40 minutes, then remove from
  the oven, allow to cool and slice into strips.*
- *Heat the extra-virgin olive oil in a wok and stir-fry the
  onion and garlic for 2–3 minutes.*
- *Add the lemongrass, chilli, ginger and tamarind paste.*
- *Add the peppers and mangetout and stir-fry for a
  further 2 minutes.*
- *Stir in the coconut milk and chicken, and simmer
  gently for 10 minutes, then serve immediately.
  Season to taste with freshly ground black pepper.*

*Carbohydrate content per serving: **17** grams*

Chicken chop suey

Once again, poultry with peppers is virtually the perfect nutritional and gastronomic combination, providing most of our essential nutritional requirements. And again, the perfect combination of healthy nutritious food only takes minutes to prepare and cook.

For 2
- 3 tbsp extra-virgin olive oil
- 200 grams skinless chicken breast, sliced into thin strips
- 1 tsp sesame oil
- 1 garlic clove, peeled and finely chopped
- 1 slice fresh ginger root, peeled and finely chopped
- 75 grams spring onions, chopped into 4–5 cm lengths
- 1 small yellow pepper, deseeded and sliced
- 1 small red pepper, deseeded and sliced
- 75 grams mangetout
- 2 tbsp light soy sauce
- 2 tbsp sweet sherry
- 100 grams beansprouts
- Freshly ground black pepper

- *Heat 2 tbsp extra-virgin olive oil in the wok and stir-fry the chicken strips for 3–4 minutes.*
- *Remove from the wok with a perforated spoon, set aside and cover.*
- *Heat the remaining olive oil and the sesame oil, and sauté the garlic, ginger and spring onions for 1–2 minutes.*
- *Add the peppers, mangetout, soy sauce, sherry and beansprouts. Season to taste, and stir-fry for 2–3 minutes.*

- *Return the chicken to the wok and cook over medium heat for a final 2–3 minutes, and serve immediately.*

Carbohydrate content per serving: **8** *grams*

Duck with plum sauce

Kale is one of the richest sources of the natural antioxidant vitamin C.

For 2
3 tbsp extra-virgin olive oil
300 grams duck breast, cubed
4 shallots, peeled and chopped
1 garlic clove, peeled and chopped
3 slices fresh root ginger, peeled and chopped
75 grams button mushrooms, halved
75 grams kale, roughly chopped
1 tbsp dry sherry
2 tbsp plum sauce
50 ml chicken stock
1 tbsp chopped fresh coriander
Freshly ground black pepper

- *Heat the extra-virgin olive oil in a wok and stir-fry the duck breast for 3–4 minutes, then remove the duck breast from the wok with a perforated spoon and set aside.*
- *Add the shallots, garlic, ginger, mushrooms and kale to the wok and stir-fry for 2–3 minutes, then add the sherry, plum sauce and chicken stock.*
- *Return the duck breast to the wok, stir in the coriander and stir-fry for a final 3–4 minutes.*
- *Season to taste and serve immediately.*

Carbohydrate content per serving: **12** *grams*

Turkey in cherry tomato and chilli sauce
Chillies are actually members of the pepper (or capsicum)
family and provide a rich source of vitamins A and C as well
as the mineral iron.

For 2
2 tbsp extra-virgin olive oil
250 grams turkey breast fillets, sliced into thin strips
2 tbsp tomato purée
10 cherry tomatoes, halved
1 large red chilli, deseeded and finely chopped
50 ml chicken stock
1 tbsp chopped fresh oregano (or 2 tsp dried
  oregano)
100 grams wild rocket

- *Heat the extra-virgin olive oil in a wok, then stir-fry the
  sliced turkey for 3–4 minutes.*
- *Stir in the tomato purée, cherry tomatoes, chilli and
  chicken stock.*
- *Add the fresh (or dried) oregano.*
- *Simmer gently for 7–8 minutes, then serve on a bed
  of wild rocket.*

*Carbohydrate content per serving: **9** grams*

Balti chicken
Cooking does not have to follow strict rules. This recipe combines Indian spices with chicken and oyster sauce with vegetables. It can be cooked in less than 15 minutes and tastes delicious.

For 2
2 tbsp Schwartz balti crushed curry spices
4 tbsp extra-virgin olive oil
150–200 grams chicken breast, sliced into thin strips
2 spring onions, chopped into 3–4 cm lengths on the diagonal
2 garlic cloves, peeled and finely chopped
3 large courgettes, chopped lengthways
1 medium green pepper, deseeded and sliced into thin strips
3 slices root ginger, peeled and finely chopped
1 tbsp oyster sauce
50 ml water
Freshly ground black pepper

- *Dry stir-fry the spices for 1 minute in a wok, then remove from the wok and set aside.*
- *Heat 2 tbsp of extra-virgin olive oil in the wok and stir-fry the chicken for 3–4 minutes.*
- *Stir in the spices and stir-fry for a further 1–2 minutes.*

At the same time
- *Heat the remaining olive oil in a separate frying pan and stir-fry the spring onions, garlic, courgettes, pepper and ginger for 3–4 minutes.*
- *Stir in the oyster sauce and water, and heat gently for a further minute.*
- *Serve the vegetables with the chicken and season to taste.*

Carbohydrate content per serving: **6** *grams*

Meat

Grilled pepper steak with French beans

For 2   2 sirloin or fillet steaks, about 150 grams each, and no
more than 2.5 cm thick
2 tbsp extra-virgin olive oil
Freshly ground black pepper
100 grams French beans

- *Brush the steaks with olive oil on both sides and season liberally with freshly ground black pepper.*
- *Place under a hot grill, at least 8 cm from the source of heat, and grill to taste, turning once.*
- *Steam the French beans until tender but still firm. The French beans can be simply served with the steaks or with one of the sauces below.*

Carbohydrate content per serving: negligible

. . . .

Garlic butter sauce

75 grams unsalted butter
2 garlic cloves, peeled and grated
1 tsp chopped flat-leaf parsley
1 tsp lemon juice
Freshly ground black pepper

- *Heat the butter in a small saucepan, stir in the garlic, parsley, lemon juice and freshly ground black pepper, and serve.*

*Carbohydrate content per serving: **2** grams*

Beef kebabs

For 2   250 grams lean steak, cubed
1 large red pepper, deseeded and chopped into 3 cm
   cubes
12 button mushrooms, wiped and trimmed
1 large green pepper, deseeded and chopped into
   3 cm cubes
12 baby yellow squash
Freshly ground black pepper
3 tbsp extra-virgin olive oil
2 tbsp chopped fresh chives, to garnish

Marinade

2 tbsp dry sherry
1 tbsp light soy sauce
1 garlic clove, peeled and finely chopped
1 slice of fresh ginger root, peeled and finely chopped
1 tsp freshly squeezed lemon juice
1 tsp honey
Pinch of rock salt
Freshly ground black pepper

- *Marinate the steak for 2–3 hours. Soak the wooden skewers in water for a similar period.*
- *Thread the steak, peppers, button mushrooms and squash on the skewers. Brush with extra-virgin olive oil and season with freshly ground black pepper, then grill (or barbecue) until the meat is cooked to taste.*
- *Garnish with chopped fresh chives, and serve with a crispy green salad (see page 79).*

*Carbohydrate content per serving: **13** grams (including salad)*

Moussaka

For 2   1 large fresh aubergine, sliced
Pinch of rock salt
3 tbsp extra-virgin olive oil
1 large onion, peeled and finely chopped
1 medium garlic clove, peeled and finely chopped
250 grams beef mince
3 large plum tomatoes, peeled and chopped
1 tbsp tomato purée
75 ml beef stock
Freshly ground black pepper

Sauce   15 grams butter
15 grams plain flour
150 ml full-cream milk
50 grams grated cheese (preferably, but not
    essentially, Greek Kefalotyri)
Freshly ground black pepper

- *Clean and slice the aubergine, then arrange in salted layers in a colander for 30 minutes. Rinse thoroughly and pat dry.*
- *Arrange the aubergine slices in a single layer on a baking tray, brush with a thin layer of olive oil and cook in a pre-heated oven at 180°C (gas mark 4) for 10 minutes. Remove from the oven and set aside to cool.*
- *Heat 2 tbsp of the olive oil and sauté the onion and garlic for 1–2 minutes until soft, then add the minced beef, stirring regularly until evenly browned. Add the chopped tomatoes and tomato purée, and stir in the stock. Season to taste and gently simmer for 10–15 minutes.*
- *Arrange half the aubergine slices in the base of an ovenproof casserole dish, add the beef mixture, then top with a second layer of aubergine slices.*

- *To prepare the sauce, heat the butter in a saucepan until melted, remove from the heat and gradually mix in the flour, stirring constantly. Return to a low heat and slowly add the milk, stirring constantly. When the mixture has reached an even consistency, add the grated cheese and stir until evenly melted into the sauce. Season to taste.*
- *Pour the sauce over the mixture in the casserole dish, top with a little grated cheese and bake in a preheated oven for 35–40 minutes at 180°C (gas mark 4).*
- *Serve with Feta and olive salad (see page 71).*

*Carbohydrate content per serving: **27** grams (including salad)*

. . . .

Sirloin steak with Stilton cheese

For 2   2 sirloin steaks, about 150 grams each
2 tbsp extra-virgin olive oil
50 grams Stilton cheese, crumbled
Pinch of rock salt
Freshly ground black pepper
1 tsp chopped fresh chives, to garnish

- *Brush the steaks with olive oil, then grill under medium heat according to individual taste (3–4 minutes per side is usually adequate).*
- *Season to taste, top with crumbled Stilton cheese, then place under the grill until the cheese melts.*
- *Serve immediately, garnished with freshly chopped chives.*

Carbohydrate content per serving: negligible

Sliced beef in oyster sauce

This dish will have a better aesthetic appearance if you use a mixture of different mushrooms, but the nutritional value is the same whichever you use.

For 2
250 grams steak, sliced into thin strips
3 tbsp extra-virgin olive oil
1 garlic clove, peeled and finely chopped
2 slices fresh ginger root, peeled and finely chopped
100 grams mushrooms, wiped and halved
4 spring onions, chopped into 3–4 cm lengths
100 grams broccoli florets
1 small red pepper, deseeded and finely sliced
½ tsp granulated sugar
Freshly ground black pepper
1 green chilli, deseeded and cut into strips, to garnish (optional)

Marinade
1 tbsp light soy sauce
1 tbsp oyster sauce
1 tbsp sweet sherry
1 tsp cornflour

- *Mix the soy sauce, oyster sauce, sherry and cornflour to an even consistency, then add to the sliced beef in a large bowl. Marinate in the fridge for 3–4 hours.*
- *Heat 2 tbsp of the extra-virgin olive oil in the wok and stir-fry the beef for 2 minutes.*
- *Add the ginger and garlic and cook for a further 2 minutes, stirring constantly. Remove from the wok with a perforated spoon and set aside.*
- *Heat the remaining olive oil in the wok, add the mushrooms, broccoli, spring onions and red pepper, and stir-fry for 2–3 minutes.*

- *Return the beef to the wok, add the oyster sauce marinade and sugar, and stir-fry for a further 2–3 minutes.*
- *Season with freshly ground black pepper and serve garnished with green chilli strips.*

Carbohydrate content per serving: 16 grams

....

Steak with cherry tomatoes, basil and coriander

This meal provides vitamin A from tomatoes and even more antioxidants from basil and coriander.

For 2   2 tbsp extra-virgin olive oil
         250 grams minute steak
         Cherry tomatoes with basil and coriander (page 69)
         Freshly ground black pepper

- *Heat the extra-virgin olive oil in a large frying pan and fry the minute steak for 3–4 minutes, turning once.*

At the same time
- *Cook the cherry tomatoes with basil and coriander.*

- *Season to taste and serve immediately.*

Carbohydrate content per serving: 4 grams

Sweet and sour pork

For 2
2 tbsp plain flour
Pinch of rock salt
Freshly ground black pepper
250 grams lean pork fillet, sliced thinly on the
    diagonal
3 tbsp extra-virgin olive oil
4 spring onions, chopped into 4–5 cm lengths
1 garlic clove, peeled and finely chopped
1 small red pepper, deseeded and finely sliced
1 small yellow pepper, deseeded and finely sliced
1 tsp granulated sugar
10 ml white wine vinegar
50 ml pork stock
1 tsp tomato purée
1 tbsp light soy sauce
1 tbsp sweet sherry
Finely chopped spring onion, to garnish

- *Coat the pork with seasoned flour.*
- *Heat 2 tbsp of the olive oil in the wok and stir-fry the pork over a medium heat for 4–5 minutes, stirring frequently.*
- *Remove the pork with a perforated spoon, set aside and cover.*
- *Heat the remaining tbsp of olive oil in the wok. Reduce the heat to medium and sauté the spring onions and garlic for about a minute, then add the red and yellow peppers, and stir-fry for 2–3 minutes.*
- *Return the pork to the wok, stir in the sugar, white wine vinegar, stock, tomato purée, soy sauce and sherry.*
- *Simmer for about 3–4 minutes and serve immediately, garnished with finely chopped spring onion.*

Carbohydrate content per serving: **21** *grams*

Pork with ginger

For 2   250 grams lean pork fillet, sliced thinly on the diagonal
3 tbsp extra-virgin olive oil
1 garlic clove, peeled and finely chopped
3 slices of fresh ginger root, peeled and finely
   chopped
100 grams mangetout
3 spring onions, chopped into 4–5 cm lengths
1 medium carrot, peeled and julienned
Pinch of rock salt
Freshly ground black pepper

Marinade

2 tbsp light soy sauce
1 tsp cornflour
2 tbsp dry sherry

- *Mix the soy sauce and sherry in a large bowl and stir in the cornflour to ensure an even consistency. Add the pork and marinate in the fridge for at least 2 hours.*
- *Heat 2 tbsp of the olive oil in a wok and stir-fry the pork for 2–3 minutes, stirring frequently. Remove the pork with a perforated spoon, set aside and cover.*
- *Heat the remaining tbsp of olive oil in the wok, add the garlic, ginger, mangetout, spring onions and carrot.*
- *Season to taste, stir-fry for 2–3 minutes, then return the pork to the wok. Cook for another 2 minutes and serve immediately.*

*Carbohydrate content per serving: **10** grams*

Lamb curry with red pepper

For 2   4 tbsp extra-virgin olive oil
2 medium onions, peeled and chopped
1 garlic clove, peeled and finely chopped
2 small red peppers, deseeded and finely sliced
1 bay leaf
2 green cardamom pods
350 grams lean lamb fillet, cubed
1 tsp garam masala
1 slice fresh ginger root, peeled and finely chopped
1 green chilli, deseeded and finely chopped
1 tbsp freshly squeezed lemon juice
200 gram tin of chopped plum tomatoes (not drained)
200 ml lamb stock
4 tbsp natural yoghurt
1 tbsp fresh coriander, finely chopped
Pinch of rock salt
Freshly ground black pepper
Fresh coriander leaves and slices of red chilli, to garnish

- *Heat the extra-virgin olive oil in a large, deep frying pan and sauté the onions, garlic, red peppers, bay leaf and cardamom pods for 1–2 minutes.*
- *Add the lamb and sauté for a further 4–5 minutes.*
- *Stir in the garam masala, ginger, chilli, lemon juice and tomatoes, and cook for 2–3 minutes. Stir in the stock and simmer gently for 45 minutes.*
- *Remove the bay leaf and cardamom pods, then stir in the yoghurt gradually over low heat.*
- *Finally, add the fresh coriander, season to taste and simmer over low heat for a further 3–4 minutes.*
- *Serve immediately, garnished with fresh coriander leaves and finely sliced red chilli.*

*Carbohydrate content per serving: **16** grams*

Honey-glazed pork
How simple can it be to produce a delicious meal which is both highly nutritious and cooks in less than 15 minutes? Mustard and honey are a delightful combination, complemented by the addition of a smooth, dry white wine.

For 2   2 lean pork fillets (approx 150 grams each)
Lime zest, to garnish
Red lettuce salad (page 74)

Marinade
1 tbsp Dijon mustard
1 tbsp clear honey
1 tbsp dry white wine
Pinch of cayenne pepper
Pinch of rock salt

- *Mix together the ingredients of the marinade thoroughly, and coat the pork fillets.*
- *Marinate the pork in the fridge for 3–4 hours, then place under a hot grill, about 8 cm from the heat, and cook for 10 minutes, turning 3–4 times.*
- *Garnish with lime zest and serve with red lettuce salad.*

*Carbohydrate content per serving: **23** grams*

Chilli lamb

For 2   250 grams lean lamb fillets, sliced into thin strips
3 tbsp extra-virgin olive oil
1 tsp sesame oil
1 small red chilli, deseeded and finely chopped
3 spring onions, chopped into 4–5 cm lengths
2 slices of fresh ginger root, peeled and grated
1 garlic clove, peeled and finely chopped
1 small red pepper, deseeded and finely sliced
1 small orange pepper, deseeded and finely sliced
50 grams sugarsnap peas
2 tbsp light soy sauce
2 green courgettes, chopped on the diagonal
Freshly ground black pepper
Pinch of rock salt

- *Heat 2 tbsp of the olive oil in a wok and stir-fry the lamb until tender. Remove from the pan with a perforated spoon, pat dry and set aside to cool.*
- *Heat the remaining olive oil and sesame oil in the wok, add the chilli, spring onions, ginger, garlic, peppers, sugarsnap peas and soy sauce, and stir-fry for 1–2 minutes.*
- *Return the lamb to the wok, add the courgettes, season to taste, stir-fry for a further 2–3 minutes and serve.*

*Carbohydrate content per serving: **7** grams*

Baked Bolognese peppers
Parmesan cheese tops this delicious and superbly nutritious
dish perfectly, adding a healthy helping of vitamin D.

For 4 2 tbsp extra-virgin olive oil
2 medium red onions, peeled and diced
2 garlic cloves, peeled and finely chopped
300 grams lean minced beef
1 tbsp tomato purée
4 large vine-ripened tomatoes, peeled and diced (or a
    400 gram tin of plum tomatoes, drained before use)
1 tbsp chopped fresh oregano
Freshly ground black pepper
4 large red peppers, deseeded and tops removed
Freshly grated Parmesan cheese
Fresh oregano, to garnish

- *Heat the extra-virgin olive oil in a frying pan and sauté the onion and garlic for 1–2 minutes.*
- *Add the mince and stir until browned.*
- *Mix in the tomato purée, tomatoes and oregano, season to taste and gently simmer for 6–8 minutes.*
- *Spoon the mixture into the peppers and place the peppers on a baking tray, adding a little water to the tray.*
- *Cook in the centre of a preheated oven at 160°C (gas mark 2) for 30–35 minutes.*
- *Remove from the oven, and sprinkle freshly grated Parmesan cheese over the peppers.*
- *Grill under a medium grill until the cheese melts, garnish with fresh oregano and serve immediately with semi-dried tomatoes with herbs (page 69).*

*Carbohydrate content per serving: **17** grams*

Beefburgers with herbs

There is no such thing as a boring hamburger! The potential variations are almost infinite. You can use beef, lamb, pork or turkey mince, and vary the herbs (or omit them) according to taste. The only part you definitely leave out on a low-carbohydrate diet is the bun – and as that has the least taste, it's the least important.

For 2   250 grams lean mince
1 small red onion, finely diced
1 small garlic clove, finely chopped
1 tbsp chopped fresh basil
1 tsp chopped fresh coriander
1 tsp Worcestershire sauce
1 medium free-range egg, beaten
Pinch of rock salt
Freshly ground black pepper
2 tbsp extra-virgin olive oil
Green salad with herbs (page 74)

- *Mix together the mince, onion, garlic, basil, coriander, Worcestershire sauce and egg in a large mixing bowl, preferably by hand (definitely the best way for making hamburgers), and season to taste.*
- *Divide into 4 roughly equal pieces, then roll each into a ball and pat gently to slightly flatten.*
- *Chill in the fridge for 1–2 hours.*
- *Heat the olive oil in a medium frying pan, and cook the hamburgers for about 8 minutes (but vary according to individual taste), turning once.*
- *Serve immediately with green salad with herbs.*

*Carbohydrate content per serving: **2** grams (without salad); **3** grams (with salad)*

Stir-fried chilli beef
The Szechuan pepper in Chinese five-spice is not a pepper,
but rather the berries of a prickly ash tree, and chilli is actually
a member of the pepper family. Confused? No matter – just
enjoy this delicious dish!

For 2
200 grams lean beef fillet, thinly sliced
4 tbsp extra-virgin olive oil
1 tsp sesame oil
3 spring onions, chopped into 3–4 cm lengths
1 garlic clove, peeled and finely chopped
3 slices of fresh ginger root, peeled and finely
  chopped
1 green chilli, deseeded and finely chopped
1 medium yellow pepper, deseeded and thinly sliced
1 medium red pepper, deseeded and thinly sliced
75 grams mangetout
75 grams broccoli florets
1 tsp ground Chinese five-spice
50 grams beansprouts
Pinch of rock salt
Freshly ground black pepper
Fresh basil and coriander leaves, to garnish

Marinade
2 tbsp light soy sauce
2 tbsp sweet sherry
1 tsp cornflour
1 garlic clove, peeled and finely chopped

- *Mix together the ingredients of the marinade, and
  marinate the beef strips for 3–4 hours.*
- *Heat 2 tbsp of extra-virgin olive oil in a wok and stir-
  fry the beef for about 2 minutes.*

- *Remove from the wok with a perforated spoon and set aside.*
- *Heat the remaining olive oil and sesame oil, then sauté the spring onions, garlic, ginger and chilli for 1–2 minutes.*
- *Add the peppers, mangetout, broccoli and Chinese five-spice, and stir-fry for 2 minutes.*
- *Return the beef to the wok, add the beansprouts and the remainder of the marinade, season to taste, then stir-fry for a final 2–3 minutes.*
- *Serve immediately, garnished with fresh basil and coriander leaves.*

*Carbohydrate content per serving: **8** grams*

Beef jalfrezi curry with peppers

For 2
5 tbsp extra-virgin olive oil
250 grams minute steak, thinly sliced
1 tsp black mustard seeds
1 tsp cumin seeds
1 medium red onion, peeled and chopped
1 medium garlic clove, peeled and finely chopped
1 tbsp medium curry powder
2 tsp plain flour
75 ml beef stock
3 slices fresh ginger root, peeled and finely chopped
1 medium red pepper, deseeded and finely sliced
1 medium green pepper, deseeded and finely sliced
1 tbsp chopped fresh coriander
Freshly ground black pepper
100 grams wild rocket leaves

- *Heat 2 tbsp extra-virgin olive oil in a large frying pan and stir-fry the steak for 3–4 minutes, then remove from the pan and set aside.*
- *Wipe the pan dry then stir-fry the mustard and cumin seeds, then remove from the pan and set aside.*
- *Add the remaining olive oil to the pan and sauté the onion and garlic for 3–4 minutes.*
- *Remove from the heat, stir in the curry powder and flour, then gradually stir in the stock.*
- *Return the steak to the pan, stir in the ginger, peppers, coriander, mustard and cumin seeds, and simmer gently for 4–5 minutes.*
- *Season to taste and serve immediately with wild rocket.*

*Carbohydrate content per serving: **12** grams*

Parma ham and Parmesan frittata

Parma ham is a rich source of essential amino acids and vitamins, especially thiamin (vitamin B$_1$), which combines perfectly, both gastronomically and nutritionally, with the taste (and vitamin D) of Parmesan and eggs.

For 2
4 large free-range eggs, beaten
1 large plum tomato, peeled and chopped
2 tsp chopped fresh oregano
100 grams Parma ham, finely chopped
50 grams Parmesan cheese, grated
Pinch of rock salt
Freshly ground black pepper
2 tbsp extra-virgin olive oil
2 spring onions, finely chopped
1 garlic clove, peeled and finely chopped
Red lettuce salad (page 74)

- *Mix together the eggs, tomato, oregano, Parma ham and Parmesan cheese, reserving some cheese to garnish, and season to taste.*
- *Heat the extra-virgin olive oil in a medium frying pan, and gently sauté the spring onions and garlic for 2–3 minutes.*
- *Add the egg mixture and cook over low heat for about 10 minutes, until almost set.*
- *Garnish with freshly grated Parmesan, and place under a low grill for 1–2 minutes.*
- *Serve with red lettuce salad.*

*Carbohydrate content per serving: **3** grams (without salad); **14** grams (with salad)*

Sesame beef with ginger and lemongrass

Sesame seeds provide the essential omega-6 fatty acids in our diet.

For 2
4 tbsp extra-virgin olive oil
250 grams minute steak, sliced into strips
4 slices fresh root ginger, peeled and chopped
2 stalks lemongrass, dehusked and finely chopped
1 tbsp sesame seeds
75 grams carrot, peeled and sliced julienne
75 grams mangetout
1 small red chilli, deseeded and finely chopped
1 medium red pepper, deseeded and finely sliced
1 tbsp chopped fresh chives, to garnish

- *Heat 2 tbsp of the extra-virgin olive oil in a medium frying pan and gently stir-fry the minute steak for 2–3 minutes.*
- *Add the ginger, lemongrass and sesame seeds, and stir-fry for a further 3-4 minutes.*

At the same time
- *Heat the remaining 2 tbsp of olive oil in a wok and stir-fry the carrot, mangetout, chilli and pepper for 3–4 minutes.*

- *Serve the sesame beef with the vegetables, garnished with chopped chives.*

*Carbohydrate content per serving: **9** grams*

Meatballs with tomato and basil sauce
Tomatoes are a rich source of the important antioxidant lycopene, which clears free radicals and helps to prevent the ageing process.

For 2	250 grams lean minced beef
	1 medium red onion, peeled and finely diced
	1 garlic clove, peeled and finely chopped
	1 egg, beaten
	2 tbsp chopped fresh basil leaves
	Tomato sauce (page 214)
	100 grams French beans
	100 grams yellow baby squash, halved
	Freshly ground black pepper
	1 tbsp chopped chives (optional)

- *Mix together the mince, onion, garlic, egg, and 1 tbsp of chopped fresh basil in a medium mixing bowl.*
- *Form the mixture into small balls, 3–4 cm in diameter.*
- *Place on a baking tray and cook under a hot grill (approx 8–10 cm from the grill) for about 8 minutes, turning 2–3 times.*

At the same time
- *Make the tomato sauce.*
- *Lightly steam the French beans and yellow squash for 10 minutes or microwave the vegetables for 3–4 minutes.*
- *Serve the meatballs, spoon over some tomato sauce, and add the vegetables.*
- *Season to taste and garnish with chopped chives.*

*Carbohydrate content per serving: **12** grams (only **6** grams without tomato sauce)*

Spaghetti Bolognese

Red meat is not essential for this most Italian of classical dishes. Turkey mince is very nutritious and low in saturated fats – or vegetarian mince can be substituted for the turkey mince, and vegetable stock for the chicken stock for vegetarians.

For 2
3 tbsp extra-virgin olive oil
1 medium red onion, peeled and chopped
2 garlic cloves, peeled and finely chopped
200 grams turkey mince (or vegetarian substitute)
1 tbsp tomato purée
150 ml chicken stock
1 tbsp chopped fresh basil leaves (or 1 tsp dried basil)
Freshly ground black pepper
40 grams wholemeal spaghetti

- *Heat the extra-virgin olive oil in a medium frying pan.*
- *Sauté the onion and garlic for 2–3 minutes.*
- *Add the turkey mince and stir regularly until browned.*
- *Stir in the tomato purée, stock and basil, season to taste and simmer gently for 5–7 minutes.*

At the same time
- *Cook the spaghetti.*

- *When cooked, put the spaghetti in serving dishes and pour the sauce on top.*

*Carbohydrate content per serving: **20 grams***

Chilli con carne
This recipe is equally suitable for vegetarians by substituting turkey mince with vegetarian mince, and chicken stock with vegetable stock. It is just as delicious without the chilli for those averse to hot dishes.

For 2   30 grams dried red kidney beans (or 50 grams tinned red kidney beans)
2 tbsp extra-virgin olive oil
1 medium red onion, peeled and chopped
200 grams turkey mince
1 level tbsp wholemeal flour
½ tsp chilli powder (optional)
1 tbsp tomato purée
200 ml chicken stock
50 grams wholegrain rice

* *Place the dried kidney beans in a medium saucepan, cover with cold water and bring to the boil for 15 minutes, then remove from the heat and allow to cool for at least 1 hour.*
* *Drain the cooked (or tinned) beans.*
* *Heat the extra-virgin olive oil in a medium frying pan and sauté the onion and garlic for 1–2 minutes.*
* *Add the mince and cook until brown.*
* *Stir in the flour, chilli powder and tomato purée, then gradually add the stock.*
* *Simmer gently for 10 minutes.*

At the same time
* *Cook the rice.*

* *When cooked, serve the chilli with the rice.*

Carbohydrate content per serving: **31** *grams*

Lasagne

This meal has been prepared for four rather than two persons simply because we are constrained by the predetermined shape of the commercial sheets of lasagne. Of course, home-made lasagne can be easily made in smaller sizes and shapes.

For 4   Bolognese sauce (see page 139, but make enough
          for 4 servings)
          30 grams unsalted butter
          30 grams plain flour
          150 ml milk
          4 sheets of dried lasagne
          1 tbsp freshly grated Parmesan cheese
          100 grams fresh watercress
          Balsamic vinegar
          Freshly ground black pepper

- *Melt the butter in a medium saucepan, then remove from the heat and stir in the flour until the mixture is smooth.*
- *Return the pan to a gentle heat and gradually add the milk, stirring constantly, until the sauce just begins to thicken.*
- *Remove from the heat, continuing to stir.*
- *Using a roasting tin of approximately the same dimensions as the sheets of lasagne, spread about a quarter of the Bolognese sauce over the base of the tin, top with about a fifth of the white sauce, then cover with a sheet of lasagne.*
- *Repeat this three times, then cover the final sheet of lasagne with the remaining white sauce, sprinkle over the grated Parmesan cheese and cook in the centre*

of a preheated oven at 180°C (gas mark 4) for 30
minutes.
* *Divide the lasagne into four equal portions and serve
immediately with fresh watercress.*
* *Drizzle a little balsamic vinegar over the watercress
and season to taste.*

*Carbohydrate content per serving: **20** grams*

Shellfish

Chilli tiger prawns with mangetout

For 2
2 tbsp extra-virgin olive oil
1 garlic clove, peeled and finely chopped
2 spring onions, chopped into 4–5 cm lengths
100 grams mangetout
1 small green chilli, deseeded and finely chopped
250 grams cooked tiger prawns, peeled and deveined
1 tbsp sweet sherry
Pinch of rock salt
Freshly ground black pepper
Sesame oil
Chopped fresh chives, to garnish

- *Heat the olive oil and sauté the garlic, spring onions, mangetout and chilli for about 2 minutes.*
- *Add the cooked tiger prawns and sherry. Season to taste and stir-fry for another 2 minutes, stirring frequently.*
- *Serve on warm plates, drizzle over a few drops of sesame oil and garnish with freshly chopped chives.*

Carbohydrate content per serving: 6 grams

Hot and spicy prawns

For 2

2 tbsp extra-virgin olive oil
3 spring onions, chopped into 4–5 cm lengths
1 garlic clove, peeled and finely chopped
2 tsp plain flour
100 ml fish stock
2 tsp Worcestershire sauce
2 tsp lemon juice
2 tsp tomato purée
4–5 drops of Tabasco sauce
1 bay leaf
Pinch of rock salt
Freshly ground black pepper
1 small orange pepper, deseeded and sliced
1 small yellow pepper, deseeded and sliced
1 tbsp chopped fresh coriander
250 grams cooked and peeled tiger prawns
Fresh coriander leaves, to garnish

- *Heat the extra-virgin olive oil in a wok and sauté the spring onions and garlic.*
- *Remove from the heat and stir in the flour.*
- *Gradually stir in the fish stock, then add the Worcestershire sauce, lemon juice, tomato purée, Tabasco sauce and bay leaf.*
- *Season to taste and simmer for 2–3 minutes, stirring frequently.*
- *Add the peppers, coriander and pre-cooked tiger prawns, and simmer for a further 4–5 minutes.*
- *Remove the bay leaf before serving and garnish with fresh coriander leaves.*

*Carbohydrate content per serving: **11** grams*

Scallops and asparagus with sweet chilli sauce

Scallops and asparagus complement one another wonderfully in every respect: taste, texture and nutritional content. This recipe has extra zest – and vitamins – when fresh chilli is included; however, it is still delicious and nutritious without chilli, for those who prefer life less hot!

For 2
1 bunch of fresh asparagus, trimmed and chopped into 5–6 cm lengths
3 tbsp extra-virgin olive oil
1 garlic clove, peeled and finely chopped
2 shallots, finely chopped
250 grams cleaned, fresh scallops
1 small red chilli, deseeded and finely chopped (optional)
2 tbsp light soy sauce
2 tbsp sweet sherry
½ tsp granulated sugar
30 grams melted butter
Freshly ground black pepper
Fresh coriander leaves, to garnish

- *Lightly steam the asparagus, transfer to a warm plate and cover.*
- *Heat the extra-virgin olive oil in the wok and sauté the garlic, shallots, scallops and chilli over medium heat for 3–4 minutes.*
- *Add the soy sauce, sherry, sugar and melted butter, season with freshly ground black pepper and cook for a further 2 minutes.*
- *Arrange the asparagus aesthetically on warm plates, serve the chilli scallops on the asparagus and garnish with fresh coriander leaves.*

*Carbohydrate content per serving: **4** grams*

Ginger scallops with mangetout

For 2
   3 tbsp extra-virgin olive oil
   250 grams fresh, cleaned scallops
   1 garlic clove, peeled and finely chopped
   3 slices fresh ginger root, peeled and finely chopped
   100 grams mangetout
   1 small red pepper, deseeded and finely sliced
   1 tbsp light soy sauce
   2 tbsp freshly squeezed orange juice
   Freshly ground black pepper
   Chopped fresh chives, to garnish

- *Heat the extra-virgin olive oil in the wok, add the scallops and sauté for 2–3 minutes. Remove the scallops carefully (to prevent breaking) with a perforated spoon.*
- *Add the garlic and ginger to the wok, and stir-fry for 30–40 seconds, then add the mangetout and pepper, and sauté for a further 2 minutes.*
- *Return the scallops to the wok, add the soy sauce and orange juice, stir gently and cook for a final 2–3 minutes. Serve garnished with chopped fresh chives.*

*Carbohydrate content per serving: **7** grams*

Creamy prawns with basil

Cayenne chilli originated in India (unlike other chillis which were introduced to Europe by Christopher Columbus from his travels in the west), but cayenne actually takes its name from a region of French Guyana! Confusing, but incredibly nutritious.

For 2
3 tbsp extra-virgin olive oil
1 spring onion, finely chopped
1 garlic clove, peeled and finely chopped
300 grams cooked prawns, thawed
4 tbsp water
1 tbsp dry sherry
1 tsp Dijon mustard
1 tbsp chopped fresh basil
1 tsp cornflour
100 ml single cream
Pinch of cayenne pepper
Sprigs of fresh dill, to garnish

- *Heat the extra-virgin olive oil in a wok and stir-fry the spring onion and garlic for about a minute.*
- *Add the prawns and stir-fry over medium heat for another minute.*
- *Stir in 2 tbsp water, sherry and mustard.*
- *Mix the cornflour with 2 tbsp water to a smooth paste.*
- *Remove the pan from the heat, and gradually stir in the cornflour paste.*
- *Return to the heat and simmer gently for 1–2 minutes, then stir in the cream and cayenne pepper.*
- *Heat through gently and serve immediately, garnished with sprigs of fresh dill.*

Carbohydrate content per serving: **5 grams**

Spicy tiger prawns with coconut
Prawns have a marvellous ability to absorb spicy flavours,
producing a delectable mixture of taste, texture and nutrition.

For 2   2 tsp ground cumin
         1 tsp ground turmeric
         2 tsp ground coriander
         2 tbsp extra-virgin olive oil
         1 medium onion, peeled and sliced
         1 garlic clove, peeled and finely chopped
         1 medium green chilli, deseeded and finely chopped
         10 cooked tiger prawns, heads and shells removed
         1 tbsp chopped fresh coriander
         100 ml coconut cream
         Freshly ground black pepper
         75 grams sugarsnap peas
         1 large yellow pepper, deseeded and finely sliced
         Fresh coriander leaves, to garnish

- *Dry stir-fry the cumin, turmeric and ground coriander over medium heat for about 1 minute.*
- *Add the extra-virgin olive oil and sauté the onion, garlic and chilli for 2 minutes, stirring frequently.*
- *Add the tiger prawns and stir-fry for about 2 minutes.*
- *Stir in the coconut cream and coriander, season to taste and heat through gently for 1–2 minutes.*

At the same time
- *Lightly steam the sugarsnap peas and pepper.*
- *Serve the spicy tiger prawns with the sugarsnap peas and pepper, garnished with fresh coriander leaves.*

*Carbohydrate content per serving: **14** grams*

Chilli prawns

Preparation time of 2–3 minutes. Nutritional value unbeatable!

For 2
   100 grams cooked and peeled prawns
1 large plum tomato, diced
2 spring onions, finely chopped
1 tbsp mayonnaise (page 210)
2 tsp Sharwood's hot chilli sauce
100 grams watercress
Freshly ground black pepper

- *Rinse the prawns in cold water to remove the overpowering 'salty' taste of the brine in which cooked prawns are usually sold.*
- *Drain, and pat dry with absorbent paper.*
- *Mix together the prawns, tomato, spring onions, mayonnaise and chilli sauce in a medium bowl.*
- *Serve on a bed of watercress and season to taste.*

*Carbohydrate content per serving: **3** grams*

Prawn fu-yung

Prawns, herbs, free-range eggs and sherry merge delectably together here. Sherry adds a delicious flavour to the recipe – but no alcohol! In cooking, alcohol boils at a lower temperature than water, so the alcohol evaporates, but the flavour remains.

For 2
- 3 tbsp extra-virgin olive oil
- 3 large free-range eggs, beaten
- 3 spring onions, washed and finely chopped
- ½ garlic clove, peeled and finely chopped
- 150 grams cooked prawns, peeled
- 2 tsp chopped fresh coriander leaves
- 1 tbsp dry sherry
- Freshly ground black pepper
- Pinch of paprika, to garnish

- *Heat 1 tbsp of olive oil in a wok and scramble the eggs lightly, so that they are still slightly 'runny'.*
- *Transfer to a bowl, and cover.*
- *Heat the remaining olive oil, sauté the spring onions and garlic for about a minute, then add the prawns and stir-fry for another minute.*
- *Add the sherry and coriander, season to taste, stir in the scrambled eggs and cook for another minute.*
- *Sprinkle over a pinch of paprika and serve immediately.*

*Carbohydrate content per serving: **2** grams*

Crab with crème fraîche

Crab has a very 'rich' flavour, and is certainly rich in nutrients, so only a little is necessary. The flavours of crab and herbs need only the simplicity of crème fraîche to bind them, figuratively and gastronomically!

For 2
100 grams white crab meat, pre-cooked
1 tbsp crème fraîche
1 spring onion, finely chopped
1 tsp chopped fresh basil
1 tsp chopped fresh coriander
2 tsp freshly squeezed lemon juice
Pinch of cayenne pepper
150 grams wild rocket

- *Mix together the crab, crème fraîche, spring onion, herbs, lemon juice and cayenne pepper in a medium bowl, and cool in the fridge for 1–2 hours.*
- *Serve on a base of wild rocket.*

*Carbohydrate content per serving: **4** grams (including salad)*

Tiger prawns with ginger and garlic
The nutritional value of prawns, ginger and garlic is obvious; less obvious is the nutritional importance of crème fraîche, both for providing essential nutrients like vitamin D and, equally important, to satisfy hunger and slow the digestive process – making us much less likely to needlessly 'snack' on junk food and ruin our diet.

For 2   3 tbsp extra-virgin olive oil
75 grams spring onions, finely chopped
1 garlic clove, peeled and finely chopped
3 slices fresh ginger root, peeled and finely chopped
200 grams cooked tiger prawns, shelled and deveined
1 tbsp sweet sherry
1 tbsp chopped fresh basil
Freshly ground black pepper
150 ml crème fraîche
1 tbsp chopped fresh chives, to garnish

- *Heat the extra-virgin olive oil in a wok, and lightly sauté the spring onions and garlic for 1–2 minutes.*
- *Stir in the ginger, prawns, sherry and basil, and season to taste.*
- *Stir-fry for 2–3 minutes, add the crème fraîche and gently heat through for 1–2 minutes.*
- *Serve immediately, garnished with chopped fresh chives.*

Carbohydrate content per serving: **5** *grams*

Mussels with ginger and herbs

For 2
500 grams fresh mussels, debearded and scrubbed
1 tbsp groundnut oil
2 shallots, peeled and diced
1 large garlic clove, peeled and sliced
3 slices fresh ginger root, peeled and sliced into
matchsticks
150 ml dry white wine
1 tbsp chopped flat-leaf parsley
1 tbsp ground almonds

- *Wash and scrub the mussels, discarding any that are open.*
- *Heat the groundnut oil in a medium saucepan and sauté the shallots and garlic for 1–2 minutes.*
- *Stir in the ginger, wine, parsley and almonds, then add the mussels.*
- *Bring to the boil, then cover the pan and simmer for 5–6 minutes.*
- *Serve immediately, discarding any unopened mussels.*

*Carbohydrate content per serving: **5 grams***

Tagliatelli with prawn and herb sauce
Vegetarians can simply omit the prawns to enjoy a similarly delicious meal.

For 2 25 grams unsalted butter
25 grams plain flour
150 ml milk
100 grams cooked prawns, rinsed
1 tbsp chopped fresh basil
1 tbsp chopped fresh parsley
50 grams tagliatelli
Freshly ground black pepper
1 spring onion, finely chopped

- *Melt the butter in a medium saucepan.*
- *Remove from the heat and stir in the flour.*
- *Return to a gentle heat and gradually add the milk, stirring constantly.*
- *When the mixture just begins to thicken, remove from the heat and stir in the prawns, basil and parsley.*

At the same time
- *Cook the tagliatelli al dente.*

- *Stir the sauce into the tagliatelli, season to taste with freshly ground black pepper and serve immediately, garnished with finely chopped spring onion.*

*Carbohydrate content per serving: **29** grams*

Spicy crab with mango

For 2   150 grams fresh white crab meat
1 small red chilli, deseeded and finely chopped
½ small mango, chopped into 2 cm cubes
1 tbsp fresh chopped coriander leaves
50 grams unsalted butter
100 grams fresh spinach leaves
Freshly ground black pepper
Coriander leaves, to garnish

- *Mix together the crab meat, chilli, mango and chopped coriander leaves in a medium bowl.*
- *Melt the butter in a medium saucepan and cook the spinach leaves for 1 minute, or until just beginning to soften, stirring constantly.*
- *Serve the crab mixture on a bed of wilted spinach, season to taste and garnish with fresh coriander leaves.*

*Carbohydrate content per serving: **12** grams*

Fish

Poached salmon

Whilst it is quite acceptable to grill rich oily fish, such as salmon, we prefer to retain its delicate flavour and texture by poaching or baking, which we cannot help but believe also retains the nutritional value better than the rather harsher environment of the grill tray. In any event, salmon is equally simple to cook by either method. Allow one salmon steak of about 150 grams per person.

- *In a saucepan boil sufficient water to just cover the salmon steaks, then reduce the heat to a gentle simmer.*
- *Add a pinch of salt to the water, then lay the fillets in the base of the pan gently, and cook for 4–5 minutes.*
- *Remove with a fish slice to prevent flaking of the fish, drain and serve on a warm plate with a simple sauce, such as lemon butter sauce (see below).*

In the southern hemisphere, the salmon tends to have a light texture, but a rather bland flavour, and therefore requires sauces for flavour enhancement. However, in the northern hemisphere, seafood of all varieties has strong and distinctive flavours, and sauces must be light to complement the intrinsic piquancy of the seafood. Salmon has such a rich natural flavour that it requires only the addition of freshly squeezed lemon or lime juice, or a simple lemon and herb butter sauce to complement and accentuate its unique taste to perfection. Several herbs seem to have been developed in nature essentially to accompany fresh salmon!

Lemon butter sauce
For 2   60 grams unsalted butter
Juice from ½ a freshly squeezed lemon

- *Heat the butter in a small saucepan and stir in the freshly squeezed lemon juice. Simmer for 20–30 seconds and serve over the salmon steaks.*

*Carbohydrate content per serving: **2** grams*

Lemon and dill butter sauce
For 2   60 grams unsalted butter
Juice from ½ a freshly squeezed lemon
2 tbsp chopped fresh dill

- *Prepare as above, but add 2 tbsp of chopped fresh dill with the juice of the lemon to the butter, simmer for 30 seconds and serve over the salmon steaks.*

*Carbohydrate content per serving: **2** grams*

Lemon and basil butter sauce
For 2   60 grams unsalted butter
Juice from ½ a freshly squeezed lemon
2 tbsp chopped fresh basil

- *Prepare as above, substituting 2 tbsp of chopped fresh basil leaves for the dill.*

*Carbohydrate content per serving: **2** grams*

Smoked salmon and sour cream salsa

For 2   4 leaves of radicchio lettuce, washed
         1 small smoked salmon fillet, finely sliced on the
             diagonal
         Pinch of paprika and some fresh basil leaves, to
             garnish

Sour cream salsa

         100 ml soured cream
         ½ Lebanese cucumber, peeled (cut 2 slices from the
             cucumber, then chop the remainder into small
             cubes)
         1 tbsp chopped fresh basil
         Freshly ground black pepper
         2 leaves of radicchio lettuce
         Paprika and basil leaves, to garnish

- *Mix together the soured cream, chopped cucumber and chopped basil, season with freshly ground black pepper and set aside to chill in the fridge for 1–2 hours.*
- *Arrange 2 leaves of radicchio lettuce on each plate.*
- *Place a slice of cucumber in the centre of the lettuce, and arrange several strips of smoked salmon on the cucumber slice.*
- *Spoon a tablespoon of sour cream salsa on to the smoked salmon, then add a second layer of smoked salmon and top with another spoonful of sour cream salsa.*
- *Sprinkle with a pinch of paprika and some fresh basil leaves to garnish, and serve immediately or chill in the fridge until required.*

*Carbohydrate content per serving: **3** grams*

Trout teriyaki

Teriyaki is delicious Japanese sauce, simply and quickly prepared, which perfectly complements the natural flavours of fish, meat or poultry.

For 2
2 trout fillets
3 tbsp sake (Japanese rice wine)
4 tbsp mirin (Japanese sweet wine)
5 tbsp Japanese soy sauce (shoyu), such as tamari –
   a dark soy sauce (do not use Chinese soy sauce
   – it is too strong for this recipe)
½ garlic clove, peeled and finely grated

- *Grate the garlic clove with a small ginger- or garlic-grater.*
- *Mix the sake, mirin, shoyu and garlic, place the trout fillets in a shallow baking dish and pour the marinade over the trout.*
- *Cover and chill in the fridge for 6–8 hours, basting with the marinade 2–3 times.*
- *Grill the marinated trout under a preheated grill (on high) for 3–4 minutes per side, turning once, and serve immediately.*

*Carbohydrate content per serving: **6** grams*

Tuna in dill mayonnaise with mangetout

For 2   200 gram tin of tuna in brine (or spring water), drained
1 tbsp chopped fresh dill
Freshly ground black pepper
100 grams French beans
100 grams mangetout
50 grams rocket
Parmesan shavings and fresh dill, to garnish
1 tbsp mayonnaise (page 210)

- *Steam the French beans and mangetout.*
- *Mix the mayonnaise, tuna and chopped fresh dill in a bowl and season with freshly ground black pepper.*
- *Serve with the French beans and mangetout on a base of rocket, and garnish with freshly ground black pepper, shavings of Parmesan cheese and fresh dill.*

*Carbohydrate content per serving: **6** grams*

Chilli tiger prawns

Although it is well known that chilli is a marvellous source of vitamins A and C, perhaps of less general knowledge is that it has been used for centuries to prevent blood clotting.

For 2
10 cooked tiger prawns, peeled
Lime wedges
Lime zest, to garnish

Marinade

1 garlic clove, peeled and grated
1 small red chilli, deseeded and very finely chopped
2 slices of fresh ginger root, peeled and finely chopped
2 tbsp light soy sauce
2 tbsp sweet sherry
2 tbsp extra-virgin olive oil
Juice of half a lemon, freshly squeezed
1 tsp sesame oil
Freshly ground black pepper

- *Mix together the ingredients of the marinade in a moderate-sized bowl.*
- *Shell the tiger prawns. The easiest way to shell a prawn is to remove the head and tail, break off the legs and the shell will then peel easily. Be careful to remove all of the shell; it has an awful texture!*
- *Marinate the prawns for 3–4 hours.*
- *Grill or barbecue the prawns for 2–3 minutes, turning once and basting with the marinade.*
- *Serve the chilli tiger prawns with lime wedges and garnish with lime zest.*

*Carbohydrate content per serving: **4 grams***

Calamari with basil and coriander

This recipe is another example of how quick and easy it is to produce delicious and very nutritious meals with simple – but healthy – ingredients. The secret lies in the content: food that is good for you almost always tastes good! With fresh calamari, extra-virgin olive oil, basil and coriander, it's just not possible to find any healthier foods. This is a perfect entrée.

For 2
200 grams fresh calamari tubes, chopped into
   1 cm rings
2 tbsp extra-virgin olive oil
2 tbsp freshly squeezed lemon juice
1 garlic clove, peeled and finely chopped
3 spring onions, finely chopped
1 tbsp chopped fresh basil leaves
1 tsp chopped fresh coriander leaves
Freshly ground black pepper
Fresh basil leaves, to garnish

- *Place the calamari in a saucepan of boiling water, reduce the heat and simmer for about 4–5 minutes.*
- *Set aside to cool.*
- *Mix together the extra-virgin olive oil and lemon juice, stir in the calamari, and marinate for 6–8 hours in the fridge.*
- *Prior to serving, stir in the garlic, spring onions and herbs. Season to taste, and garnish with fresh basil leaves.*

*Carbohydrate content per serving: **1** gram*

Cod kebabs with baby squash
With a little preparation of the marinade in advance, this dish is quick and nutritious – with delicious results! Vitamin A and C in pepper and squash complement the superb nutritional value of cod.

For 2   400 grams cod fillets, chopped into 2–3 cm cubes
2 tbsp extra-virgin olive oil
4 baby onions, peeled
8 yellow baby squash
8–10 button mushrooms, wiped
1 large red pepper, chopped into 2–3 cm segments
Freshly ground black pepper
Red lettuce salad (page 74)

Marinade
2 tbsp light soy sauce
1 tbsp sweet sherry
1 slice fresh ginger root, peeled and finely chopped
1 garlic clove, peeled and finely chopped

- *Marinate the cod for 2–3 hours.*

At the same time
- *Soak 6 wooden skewers in cold water before use.*

- *Thread the skewers with alternate cod cubes, onions, squash, button mushrooms and peppers.*
- *Brush with olive oil and grill under a hot grill, or barbecue, for 5–6 minutes.*
- *Serve with red lettuce salad.*

*Carbohydrate content per serving: **20** grams (including salad)*

Salmon with bok choy

Bok choy has a delightful texture and unique flavour. It complements salmon perfectly, especially with a light soy dressing. But be careful never to overcook the bok choy, or its intrinsic nutrition will be lost. Overcooking is the certain way to destroy natural nutrition in healthy food.

For 2
2 salmon steaks, about 150–175 grams each
25 grams butter, cubed
2 slices fresh ginger root, peeled and sliced julienne
2 bok choy, quartered vertically
Freshly ground black pepper
Sprigs of fresh dill, to garnish

Dressing
1 tbsp light soy sauce
1 tbsp sweet sherry
½ tsp sesame oil
½ tsp grated fresh root ginger

- *Mix together the soy sauce, sweet sherry, sesame oil and grated ginger, and set aside.*
- *Place the salmon steaks in the base of an ovenproof dish, top with ginger strips and dot with cubes of butter.*
- *Cover with pierced aluminium foil and bake in the centre of a preheated oven at 180°C (gas mark 4) for about 20 minutes, depending on the oven.*

Just before the salmon is ready
- *Lightly steam the bok choy (3–4 minutes is sufficient).*

- *Transfer the salmon to the plates with a perforated spoon.*
- *Place the cooked bok choy next to the salmon.*
- *Drizzle the dressing over the bok choy.*
- *Finally, garnish with sprigs of fresh dill.*

*Carbohydrate content per serving: **1** gram*

....

Cod with tomato and coriander salsa

For 2   2 cod steaks, approximately 150 grams each
1 tbsp extra-virgin olive oil
Tomato and coriander salsa (see page 213)
Pinch of rock salt
Freshly ground black pepper
Fresh coriander leaves, to garnish

- *Brush the cod steaks with the olive oil and grill on a high heat for 6–7 minutes, turning once.*
- *Season to taste and serve on warm plates with the tomato and coriander salsa, garnished with fresh coriander.*

*Carbohydrate content per serving: **7** grams*

Spicy Thai swordfish

Swordfish is 100 per cent essential proteins, and the ingredients in this recipe are complementary in both taste and nutrition, from the vitamin C in the lemon juice to the vitamin A in the lemongrass!

For 2   2 swordfish steaks (about 150–175 grams each)
2 tsp sesame seeds
1 bok choy, halved lengthways

Marinade
1 tbsp Thai fish sauce
1 tbsp sweet sherry
Juice of a freshly squeezed lemon
1 large garlic clove, peeled and finely chopped
3 slices fresh ginger root, peeled and finely chopped
1 green chilli, deseeded and finely chopped
1 stick of lemongrass, outer leaves removed, and finely chopped
1 tbsp chopped fresh coriander
1 tbsp chopped fresh Thai sweet basil

- *Mix together the ingredients of the marinade.*
- *Marinate the swordfish steaks for about 1 hour, turning once.*
- *Dry stir-fry the sesame seeds for about a minute.*
- *Steam the marinated swordfish for 5–6 minutes.*

At the same time
- *Lightly steam the bok choy for 3–4 minutes.*

- *Serve the swordfish steaks with lightly steamed bok choy and garnish with lightly toasted sesame seeds.*

*Carbohydrate content per serving: **4 grams***

Salmon steaks with herbs

This dish combines the superbly nutritious qualities of salmon with the antioxidants in herbs. (Incidentally, tarragon can also be used to treat snakebite – according to the ancient Romans!)

For 2
- 2 tbsp extra-virgin olive oil
- 2 salmon steaks, approximately 150–175 grams each
- Pinch of rock salt
- Freshly ground black pepper
- 1 tbsp chopped fresh tarragon
- 1 tbsp chopped fresh chives
- 1 tbsp freshly squeezed lemon juice
- Sprigs of fresh tarragon, to garnish
- Lemon wedges
- Char-grilled vegetables with sesame seeds (page 172)

- *Place the salmon steaks on individual sheets of aluminium foil and brush with extra-virgin olive oil.*
- *Season to taste and sprinkle the herbs evenly over the salmon.*
- *Close the foil parcels and cook in the centre of a preheated oven at 180°C (gas mark 4) for about 20 minutes, depending on the oven.*
- *Remove the salmon from the parcels, drizzle over freshly squeezed lemon juice and garnish with sprigs of fresh tarragon.*
- *Serve immediately with lemon wedges and char-grilled vegetables with sesame seeds.*

*Carbohydrate content per serving: **13** grams (**1** gram without vegetables)*

Char-grilled basil pesto salmon with asparagus
Pine nuts (in basil pesto sauce) are an excellent source of
vitamin B$_1$ and vitamin E.

For 2   1 tbsp extra-virgin olive oil

2 medium salmon fillets or steaks (approximately
150 grams each)

2 tbsp basil pesto sauce, either commercial or home-
made (page 209)

8 asparagus spears

50 grams unsalted butter

2 tbsp freshly squeezed lemon juice

Freshly ground black pepper

- *Brush the salmon fillets (or steaks) with a little extra-virgin olive oil, then grill under a hot grill (no closer than 8–10 cm from the grill).*
- *Coat one side of the salmon with the basil pesto sauce then char-grill for another 2 minutes.*

At the same time
- *Place the asparagus in the base of a suitable microwave-safe container, arranged with the thick stalks to the outside of the dish and the thin tops facing inwards.*
- *Add 2 tbsp water, cover and cook on 'high' for 2–3 minutes, then allow to stand for 1 minute.*

Or
- *Lightly steam the asparagus for 10–12 minutes.*

Then
- *Heat the butter in a small saucepan, then stir in the lemon juice.*

- *Serve the salmon with the asparagus, drizzle the lemon butter sauce over the asparagus and season with freshly ground black pepper.*

Carbohydrate content per serving: 4 grams

Char-grilled tuna steaks

Simply delicious and totally nutritious! This has to be the ultimate 10-minute meal – and so healthy. Char-grilled tuna can be served with a salad, as suggested, or with either lightly steamed or stir-fried vegetables. Tuna is usually served rare, but can be cooked for longer if you prefer.

For 2 3 tbsp extra-virgin olive oil
2 tuna steaks, approximately 150–175 grams each
Freshly ground black pepper
Rocket and olive salad (page 73)

- *Brush the tuna steaks with olive oil, sprinkle with freshly ground black pepper and char-grill for 5–6 minutes, turning once.*
- *Serve with rocket and olive salad.*

Carbohydrate content per serving: 1 gram (including salad!)

Chapter 9 Vegetarian meals

The Gi Bikini Diet is perfect for vegetarians because most vegetables are already low GI! Even for those who are not vegetarian, a low-GI diet is based on substituting high-GI foods with vegetables that are packed with taste and healthy nutrients, helping prevent heart disease, diabetes and some cancers. And remember that many of the recipes in earlier chapters can be simply adapted for vegetarians by replacing the animal proteins by a vegetable protein such as tofu.

Bok choy with oyster sauce
This is a simple and quick vegetable side dish that complements many main courses.

For 2   2 tbsp extra-virgin olive oil
½ tsp sesame oil
1 slice fresh ginger root, peeled and finely chopped
1 bok choy, shredded
1 tbsp oyster sauce
Freshly ground black pepper

- *Heat the extra-virgin olive oil and sesame oil in the wok and sauté the ginger and bok choy for about a minute.*
- *Stir in the oyster sauce, season to taste and stir-fry for a further 2 minutes.*

Carbohydrate content per serving: 3 grams

Chilli aubergine
Aubergines have the capacity to absorb flavours, particularly herbs and spices, better than virtually any other vegetable.

For 2
1 large aubergine, sliced
Rock salt
3 tbsp extra-virgin olive oil
2 large plum tomatoes, chopped
1 garlic clove peeled and finely chopped
1 medium green pepper, deseeded and chopped
2 spring onions, finely chopped
1 medium green chilli, deseeded and finely chopped
1 tbsp chopped fresh coriander
Freshly ground black pepper
Fresh coriander leaves, to garnish

- *Place the aubergine slices in a colander, sprinkle with salt and allow to stand for 20–30 minutes, then rinse thoroughly and pat dry.*
- *Heat 2 tbsp of extra-virgin olive oil in a large frying pan, and brown the aubergine slices.*
- *Remove the slices from the pan, dry on kitchen paper and chop into large chunks.*
- *Heat the remaining olive oil, add the tomatoes, garlic, green pepper, spring onions and chilli, and sauté for 3–4 minutes.*
- *Return the aubergine pieces to the pan, stir in the coriander, season to taste and cook over medium heat for 2–3 minutes.*
- *Serve immediately, garnished with fresh coriander leaves.*

*Carbohydrate content per serving: **5** grams*

Char-grilled vegetables with sesame seeds
Char-grilling is a very healthy method of cooking, retaining
almost all of the nutrition in the vegetables.

For 2
1 small green pepper, deseeded and quartered
lengthways
1 small red pepper, deseeded and quartered
lengthways
2 small red onions, peeled and quartered lengthways
2 large plum tomatoes, quartered lengthways
4 yellow squash, halved lengthways
2 tbsp extra-virgin olive oil
Freshly ground black pepper
1 tsp sesame seeds
Fresh basil leaves, to garnish

- *Dry stir-fry the sesame seeds for about a minute, then
  set aside.*
- *Arrange the vegetables in a single layer, skin
  uppermost, on a metal grill-tray, brush with extra-
  virgin olive oil and grill under medium heat,
  approximately 8 cm from the grill, for 7–8 minutes.*
- *Remove from the grill, and peel the skin from the
  peppers, onions and tomatoes.*
- *Season to taste, and sprinkle lightly toasted sesame
  seeds over the vegetables.*
- *Serve immediately, garnished with fresh basil leaves.*

*Carbohydrate content per serving: **12** grams*

Mushrooms with garlic
Mushrooms are a very rich source of the mineral zinc, which is essential for the production of one of the body's natural antioxidant enzymes, 'superoxide dismutase'.

For 2   3 tbsp extra-virgin olive oil
1 medium red onion, peeled and sliced
2 garlic cloves, peeled and finely chopped
200 grams button mushrooms, wiped
1 tbsp chopped fresh chives
1 tbsp chopped fresh coriander
1 tbsp freshly squeezed lemon juice
Freshly ground black pepper
Fresh coriander leaves, to garnish

- *Heat the extra-virgin olive oil in a wok and gently sauté the onion and garlic for 1–2 minutes.*
- *Add the mushrooms, and sauté for a further 3–4 minutes, stirring constantly.*
- *Stir in the chives and coriander, add the lemon juice and season to taste.*
- *Garnish with fresh coriander leaves.*

*Carbohydrate content per serving: **5** grams*

Spicy vegetables

Mangetout is a variety of pea, not bean, and provides a particularly rich source of vitamin C, in addition to potassium, calcium and phosphorus.

For 2
3 tbsp extra-virgin olive oil
1 medium red onion, peeled and sliced
1 garlic clove, peeled and finely chopped
100 grams broccoli florets
50 grams mangetout
50 grams French beans
1 tsp ground cumin
1 tsp ground fennel seeds
1 tbsp chopped fresh coriander
½ tsp garam masala
1 slice fresh ginger root, peeled and finely chopped
100 ml chicken stock
100 grams spinach, chopped
1 tbsp freshly squeezed lemon juice
1 tbsp dry sherry
Pinch of rock salt
Freshly ground black pepper

- *Heat the extra-virgin olive oil in a wok and sauté the onion and garlic for 1–2 minutes.*
- *Add the broccoli, mangetout and French beans, and stir-fry for 2–3 minutes.*
- *Stir in the cumin, fennel, coriander, garam masala and ginger, and cook for about a minute, then add the chicken stock and simmer for 4–5 minutes.*
- *Stir in the spinach, lemon juice and sherry, season to taste and simmer for a final 2 minutes before serving.*

Carbohydrate content per serving: **6** *grams*

Peperonata

For 4   3 tbsp extra-virgin olive oil
1 large red onion, peeled and chopped
1 garlic clove, peeled and finely chopped
4 medium red peppers, deseeded and finely sliced
400 gram tin plum tomatoes
1 tbsp chopped fresh basil (or 1 tsp dried basil)
1 tbsp chopped fresh parsley (optional)
Freshly ground black pepper

- *Heat the extra-virgin olive oil in a medium frying pan and sauté the onion and garlic for 1–2 minutes.*
- *Stir in the peppers and stir-fry for a further 3–4 minutes.*
- *Drain the tomatoes.*
- *Add the tomatoes, basil and parsley, and simmer gently over a low heat for 3–4 minutes.*
- *Season to taste and serve immediately.*

*Carbohydrate content per serving: **10** grams*

Vegetable goulash

Unusually, the content of the powerful antioxidant lycopene is higher in cooked tomatoes than in their fresh form.

For 2
1 tbsp extra-virgin olive oil
1 garlic clove, peeled and finely chopped
1 tbsp flour
1 tbsp ground paprika
200 ml chicken stock
400 gram tin of chopped plum tomatoes
4 baby onions, peeled
150 grams broccoli florets
150 grams carrots, peeled and julienned
100 grams cauliflower florets
1 small red pepper, deseeded and sliced
1 small green pepper, deseeded and sliced
3–4 drops Tabasco sauce
Pinch of rock salt
Freshly ground black pepper
1 tbsp chopped fresh oregano
1 tbsp chopped fresh basil
100 ml soured cream
1 tbsp chopped fresh chives, to garnish
75 grams French beans
75 grams mangetout

- *Heat the extra-virgin olive oil in a medium frying pan, and sauté the garlic for a minute.*
- *Remove from the heat and stir in the flour and paprika.*
- *Return to the heat and stir in the tomatoes and stock.*
- *Add the onions, broccoli, carrots, cauliflower, peppers and Tabasco sauce, season to taste and simmer for 5 minutes.*

- *Transfer to an oven-proof casserole dish and cook in the centre of a preheated oven at 190°C (gas mark 5) for 20–25 minutes.*
- *Stir in the oregano and basil and return to the oven for 10 minutes.*
- *Remove from the oven, stir in the soured cream lightly to achieve a 'marbled' effect and garnish with chopped chives.*
- *Serve with lightly steamed French beans and mangetout.*

*Carbohydrate content per serving: **22** grams*

• •

Asparagus with lemon butter sauce

Asparagus has been considered an aphrodisiac since Roman times!

For 2   200 grams asparagus, washed and trimmed
75 grams butter
Juice of ½ a freshly squeezed lemon
Freshly ground black pepper
Fresh basil leaves, to garnish

- *Lightly steam the asparagus.*
- *Melt the butter in a small saucepan, stir in the lemon juice and season to taste.*
- *Arrange the asparagus on warm plates, pour over the lemon butter sauce and garnish with fresh basil.*

*Carbohydrate content per serving: **4** grams*

Teriyaki tofu

This meal should be prepared the evening before use – if possible – to allow the tofu to marinate. Preparation time is minimal and the meal is ready immediately the following day.

For 2
80 grams tofu, cubed
2 tbsp sake
2 tbsp mirin (sweet rice wine)
2 tbsp shoyu (Japanese soy sauce)
2 slices fresh root ginger, peeled and finely chopped
2 spring onions, finely chopped

- *Mix together the tofu, sake, mirin, shoyu, ginger root and spring onions, and marinate in the fridge for 24 hours.*
- *Serve the following day.*

*Carbohydrate content per serving: **3** grams*

Stir-fried vegetables with black bean sauce

For 2
2 tbsp extra-virgin olive oil
4 spring onions, chopped on the diagonal
1 garlic clove, peeled and chopped
3 slices fresh root ginger, peeled and chopped
75 grams chestnut mushrooms, wiped and halved
lengthways
75 grams bean sprouts
75 grams mangetout
1 medium red pepper, deseeded and sliced
Freshly ground black pepper

Sauce
2 tsp cornflour
4 tbsp water
2 tbsp dry sherry
1 tbsp light soy sauce
2 tbsp black bean sauce

• *To make the sauce, stir the cornflour into the water in a small bowl, then stir in the other ingredients for the sauce.*
• *Heat the extra-virgin olive oil in a wok and stir-fry the spring onions, garlic, ginger, mushrooms, bean sprouts, mangetout and pepper for 2–3 minutes.*
• *Add the sauce and stir-fry for a further 3–4 minutes.*
• *Season to taste and serve immediately.*

Carbohydrate content per serving: 15 grams

Stir-fried tofu with mushrooms

For 2   150 grams tofu, chopped into 2 cm cubes

       3 tbsp extra-virgin olive oil

       75 grams mangetout

       75 grams bamboo shoots, sliced into thin strips

       75 grams button mushrooms, wiped and halved

       2 slices fresh ginger root, peeled and finely chopped

       1 tbsp sesame seeds

       Freshly ground black pepper

Marinade

       1 tsp granulated sugar

       3 tbsp light soy sauce

       3 tbsp dry sherry

- *Make the marinade by mixing the ingredients together.*
- *Rinse the chopped tofu and pat dry, put it in the marinade and leave for 6–8 hours.*
- *Heat 2 tbsp extra-virgin olive oil in a wok and stir-fry the tofu and marinade for 2–3 minutes, then remove from the wok with a perforated spoon and set aside.*
- *Heat the remaining olive oil in the wok and stir-fry the mangetout, bamboo shoots, mushrooms and ginger for 2–3 minutes, then add the tofu and stir-fry for a final 2 minutes.*
- *Dry stir-fry the sesame seeds in a small saucepan for 1 minute.*
- *Season the tofu mixture to taste and serve immediately, garnished with the toasted sesame seeds.*

*Carbohydrate content per serving: **14** grams*

Coconut okra curry

For 2
2 tbsp extra-virgin olive oil
150 grams okra, topped and tailed, and halved
  lengthways
½ tsp ground coriander
½ tsp ground turmeric
½ tsp ground cumin
1 small red chilli, deseeded and finely chopped
  (optional)
3 slices fresh ginger root, peeled and finely chopped
50 ml vegetable stock
200 ml natural yoghurt
50 ml coconut milk
1 tbsp freshly chopped coriander leaves
Freshly ground black pepper
Fresh coriander leaves, to garnish

- *Heat the extra-virgin olive oil in a medium frying pan and stir-fry the okra over a medium heat for 4–5 minutes.*
- *Stir in the ground coriander, turmeric, cumin, chilli and ginger, and stir-fry for a further minute.*
- *Add the vegetable stock and simmer gently for 8–10 minutes.*
- *Stir in the yoghurt, coconut milk and fresh coriander, season to taste and heat through gently for about 2 minutes. Do not allow to boil.*
- *Serve immediately, garnished with fresh coriander leaves.*

Carbohydrate content per serving: 9 grams

Milanese risotto

For 2   2 tbsp extra-virgin olive oil
1 small red onion, peeled and finely chopped
1 medium garlic clove, peeled and finely chopped
1 medium red pepper, deseeded and chopped
1 medium yellow pepper, deseeded and chopped
2 slices fresh ginger root, peeled and finely chopped
60 grams Arborio rice
3 tbsp dry white wine
200 ml chicken (or vegetable) stock
½ tsp saffron powder
1 tbsp freshly grated Parmesan cheese
1 tbsp fresh chopped parsley
Freshly ground black pepper

* *Heat the extra-virgin olive oil in a medium frying pan and sauté the onion, garlic and peppers for 1–2 minutes.*
* *Stir in the ginger and rice and cook for 1 minute.*
* *Add the wine and simmer gently for 1 minute.*
* *Stir in the stock and saffron powder, and simmer gently until the rice is cooked and most of the liquid is absorbed.*
* *Add the Parmesan cheese and cook for a further minute, then remove from the heat, season to taste with freshly ground black pepper and serve immediately, topped with fresh parsley.*

*Carbohydrate content per serving: **30** grams*

Fettuccine with spinach and sage

For 2   60 grams fettuccine
2 tbsp extra-virgin olive oil
3 shallots, peeled and diced
2 medium garlic cloves, peeled and finely chopped
1 tbsp unsalted butter
100 grams chopped fresh spinach leaves
1 tbsp chopped fresh sage (or basil)
1 tbsp freshly grated Pecorino cheese
Freshly ground black pepper

- *Heat the extra-virgin olive oil in a small frying pan and sauté the shallots and garlic for 1–2 minutes.*
- *Melt the butter in a medium saucepan and cook the spinach and sage (or basil) for 30–60 seconds until it just begins to soften, then remove from the heat immediately.*

At the same time
- *Cook the fettuccine al dente.*

- *Stir the shallots, garlic, spinach, sage and Pecorino cheese into the fettuccine, season with freshly ground black pepper and serve immediately.*

Carbohydrate content per serving: 25 grams

Mozzarella aubergine slices with pesto sauce

For 2   1 large aubergine, washed and finely sliced
            lengthways
         Sea salt
         3 tbsp extra-virgin olive oil
         1 medium garlic clove, peeled and finely chopped
         2 tbsp coriander pesto sauce (see page 212)
         75 grams mozzarella cheese, very finely sliced
         Freshly ground black pepper
         1 tbsp chopped fresh chives
         Fresh coriander leaves

- *Place the aubergine slices in a colander, sprinkle with salt and leave for 20–30 minutes. Rinse with cold water and pat dry.*
- *Heat the extra-virgin olive oil in a large, shallow frying pan, then lightly fry the aubergine slices and garlic for 2–3 minutes, turning once.*
- *Spoon the pesto sauce evenly on each of the aubergine slices, top with the finely sliced mozzarella and cook under a hot grill (no closer than 8–10 cm from the flame) for 3–4 minutes, or until the mozzarella just begins to 'bubble'.*
- *Serve the mozzarella aubergine slices on warmed plates, season to taste and garnish with chopped fresh chives and coriander leaves.*

*Carbohydrate content per serving: **6** grams*

Spicy carrot and coriander patties

For 2
2 large carrots, peeled and grated
2 shallots, peeled and finely chopped
2 slices fresh ginger root, peeled and grated
1 small garlic clove, peeled and grated
1 tbsp chopped fresh coriander leaves
1 tbsp freshly grated Parmesan cheese
1 tbsp Bombay crushed curry spices, bought ready-made
1 tbsp plain flour
1 medium organic free-range egg, beaten
2 tbsp extra-virgin olive oil
Pinch of rock salt
Freshly ground black pepper
100 grams wild rocket
Sprigs of fresh mint, to garnish

- *Mix together the carrots, shallots, ginger, garlic, coriander, Parmesan cheese, spices and flour in a large bowl.*
- *Stir in the beaten egg.*
- *Form the carrot mixture into small patties.*
- *Heat the extra-virgin olive oil in a large frying pan.*
- *Cook the patties for 3–4 minutes, turning once.*
- *Season to taste and serve immediately with wild rocket and sprigs of fresh mint.*

*Carbohydrate content per serving: **15** grams*

Char-grilled tofu kebabs with satay sauce

For 2   75 grams tofu, chopped into 2 cm cubes

50 grams small button mushrooms, wiped

1 small green pepper, deseeded and chopped into
2 cm cubes

1 small red pepper, deseeded and chopped into 2 cm
cubes

6 baby yellow squash, halved lengthways

Freshly ground black pepper

1 tbsp chopped fresh basil leaves

Satay sauce (page 215)

Marinade

2 tbsp soy sauce

2 tbsp dry sherry

2 slices fresh root ginger, peeled and grated

1 small garlic clove, peeled and grated

- *Mix together the ingredients of the marinade and marinate the cubed tofu for 3–4 hours.*

At the same time

- *Soak the satay sticks in cold water.*

- *Thread the tofu, mushrooms, peppers and squash alternately onto the satay sticks.*
- *Drizzle over the remaining marinade and cook under a hot grill (no closer than 8–10 cm from the grill) for 6–8 minutes, turning frequently.*
- *Season to taste, garnish with chopped fresh basil leaves and serve with satay sauce.*

Carbohydrate content per serving: **27 grams**

Lentil dhal

For 2   200 grams brown lentils
2 tbsp extra-virgin olive oil
1 medium red onion, peeled and finely chopped
1 small garlic clove, peeled and crushed
1 large green chilli, deseeded and finely chopped
½ tsp ground coriander
½ tsp ground cumin
¼ tsp chilli powder
½ tsp garam masala
¼ tsp ground turmeric
600 ml organic vegetable stock

- *Place lentils in a medium bowl, cover with cold water and allow to stand for at least 8 hours, then drain before use.*
- *Heat the extra-virgin olive oil in a medium saucepan and sauté the onion and garlic for 1–2 minutes.*
- *Stir in the chilli, coriander, cumin, chilli powder, garam masala and turmeric, and stir-fry for a further 2 minutes.*
- *Stir in the vegetable stock and lentils, and simmer gently for about 1 hour.*
- *Serve immediately.*

*Carbohydrate content per serving: **24** grams*

Nasi Goreng

For 2   60 grams Arborio rice
         25 grams unsalted butter
         2 large free-range eggs, beaten
         2 tbsp extra-virgin olive oil
         2 shallots, peeled and chopped
         1 garlic clove, peeled and chopped
         1 slice fresh ginger root, peeled and chopped
         1 medium green chilli, peeled and finely chopped
         1 medium red pepper, deseeded and finely sliced
         1 medium orange pepper, deseeded and finely sliced
         2 spring onions, chopped on the diagonal into
           2–3 cm lengths
         1 tbsp chopped fresh coriander leaves
         1 tbsp chopped fresh basil leaves
         1 tbsp soy sauce
         Freshly ground black pepper
         100 grams fresh wild rocket

- Cook the rice.

Just before the rice is cooked
- Heat the butter in a medium pan and scramble the eggs, stirring constantly, then set aside.
- Heat the extra-virgin olive oil in a wok and stir-fry the shallots, garlic, ginger, chilli, peppers, spring onions, coriander and basil for 2–3 minutes.

- Stir in the scrambled eggs, cooked rice and soy sauce, and stir-fry for a further minute.
- Season to taste and serve immediately on a bed of wild rocket.

*Carbohydrate content per serving: **30** grams*

Chapter 10 Ready meals and eating out

Ready-made meals are usually considered a real problem on any diet because they are usually loaded with calories, but that need not provide a problem with a well-planned GI diet. On this programme, it is the *content* of the food rather than the *calories* which is the most important factor. For example, a tuna sandwich may contain the same calories as a tuna mayonnaise salad lunchbox but the sandwich is high GI and the tuna mayo low GI!

Cold ready meals are best from either the local deli or the deli section of your local supermarket. Here are some tips to make sure you stay low GI.

Avoid:
- Bread, rolls, wraps, tortillas, panini, ciabatta, French bread, croissants – far too high GI at one time
- Pasta, noodle or rice salads (pasta and rice are included in moderation but commercial salads are usually comprised *mainly* of rice or pasta so they can blow the diet for the day)
- Sushi (unless it is rice-free)
- Pizza (very high GI)
- Couscous

Include:
- Cooked chicken (breast, drumsticks, wings)
- Smoked salmon
- Salads of every variety (without rice or pasta)
- Salad lunchboxes with unlimited quantities of salad and 2 tablespoons of delicious low-GI fillings, for example:
    Prawn mayonnaise
    Roasted peppers

      Various cheeses
      Eggs, with or without mayo
      Coronation chicken
      Mozzarella, tomato and basil (with balsamic vinegar)
      Tuna mayo
      Sun-dried tomatoes

- Cooked salmon fillets
- Open sandwiches (or, even better, the 'No-bread sandwiches' from Pret a Manger)
- Add dressing or mayo if you like
- *Never* use low-fat dressing or mayo because this has more sugar and is actually higher GI than the normal variety!

As you can see, most deli foods are naturally low GI so the choices are almost unlimited.

Hot ready meals can be either microwavable at home or take-away.

Microwavable meals from supermarkets

It is important to consider food in a totally different way if you intend to be healthy on ready-made meals. With a little planning ahead, you will soon realise that health and 'fast food' can easily be combined – provided it is *real* fast food. Microwavable food from supermarkets is the obvious solution. Not the usual polystyrene low-fat, low-taste variety, but rather the delicious meals that are found in other gourmet (and non-diet) sections of the store and which are actually low GI.

Remember, diet foods in the terminology of supermarkets generally means low-fat or low-calorie foods, which are almost always high in sugar and therefore high GI! And supermarket diet foods always seem to have the same bland taste. Gourmet foods, on the other hand, are exactly the opposite: they are delicious and low GI. You will find a good selection of low-GI foods where you least expect on supermarket shelves. For example, who would expect to find delicious low-GI meals in the Indian food section, but there they are – provided you know how to look and what to look for.

As a general rule, avoid the 'diet', low-fat, low-calorie section of supermarket microwavable meals because these are almost always higher GI. Go directly to the gourmet section (including Indian and Chinese cuisine), where you will find the most delicious meals which are also those with a lower GI, provided you choose carefully and read the nutrition labels. Seemingly comparable meals can have immensely different GI values. Chicken sag (a blend of spinach, tomatoes and onions, with cumin seeds and green cardamoms) is low GI with less than 15 grams of carbohydrate per 350 gram meal (or less than the amount of carbohydrate in a single slice of bread, to place this in perspective), compared to the high-GI chicken biryani with 79 grams of carbohydrate in a similar serving.

Other meals within this category can obviously be divided into those that can be included in a low-GI diet and those that can't. Once again, it must be emphasised that different outlets produce different nutritional combinations of products with similar names; for example, chicken casserole will almost certainly have different carbohydrate and protein content from different outlets. Supermarkets are constantly altering the range of microwavable foods they offer, so you may not find all of the foods in the list available at all outlets. This list is not meant to be all-inclusive but merely to demonstrate the types of meals available at any given time and to encourage you, once again, to read the nutritional information on the food label. By this simple method, you will soon discover which foods can be included and which should be excluded from your diet.

Meals which can be included in a low-GI diet

Meal	Weight (g)	Carbs (g)	Protein (g)
Paprika beef			
for 2:	550	16	82
per serving:	275	8	41
Butter chicken			
for 2:	350	20	42
per serving:	175	10	21
Chicken breast in creamy white wine and mushroom sauce			
for 2:	450	5	63
per serving:	225	3	32
Barbecue chicken wings	500	20	44
Shepherd's pie			
per serving:	200	21	11
Ready-to-roast chicken breast with cherry tomatoes and mozzarella cheese			
for 2:	510	15	97
per serving:	255	8	48
Steak in creamy green peppercorn sauce			
for 2:	400	12	56
per serving:	200	6	28

Meal	Weight (g)	Carbs (g)	Protein (g)
Salmon in creamy sauce	200	10	12
Chicken breast escalopes with smoked ham, Cheddar cheese and mushrooms			
for 2:	310	less than 1	59
per serving:	155	less than 1	30
Barbecue rack of ribs			
for 2:	360	42	43
per serving:	280	21	22
Crispy lemon chicken			
for 2:	300	45	36
per serving:	150	23	18
Italian fish bake			
for 2:	400	16	48
per serving:	200	8	24
Roast duck à l'orange			
for 2:	540	32	71
per serving:	270	16	36
Salmon in watercress sauce			
for 2:	400	12	56
per serving:	200	6	28
Salmon in creamy herb sauce with asparagus			
for 2:	370	less than 1	46
per serving:	185	less than 1	23

Meal	Weight (g)	Carbs (g)	Protein (g)
Salmon with mustard and dill sauce			
for 2:	380	15	53
per serving:	190	8	27
Char-grilled chicken with peppers, onion and cheese in tomato and basil sauce			
for 2:	470	9	61
per serving:	235	5	30
Mushroom stroganoff			
for 2:	400	45	11
per serving:	200	23	6
Ready-to-roast turkey breast			
for 5:	1250	25	238
per serving:	250	5	48
Tandoori chicken with spiced couscous			
for 2:	355	36	18
per serving:	178	18	9
Thai-style prawns with cucumber, spring onion and noodles			
for 2:	300	33	12
per serving:	150	17	6

Vegetables to accompany main meals which can be included in a low-GI diet

Meal	Weight (g)	Carbs (g)	Protein (g)
Roasted Mediterranean vegetables			
for 2:	300	20	4
per serving:	150	10	2
Carrot and swede potato mash			
for 2:	450	36	9
per serving:	225	18	5
Spinach in cream sauce with garlic and nutmeg			
for 2:	300	15	9
per serving:	150	8	5

Pasta and rice

Meal	Weight (g)	Carbs (g)	Protein (g)
Spaghetti Bolognese			
for 2:	400	51	28
per serving:	200	26	14
Beef lasagne			
for 2:	380	42	22
per serving:	190	21	11

Meal	Weight (g)	Carbs (g)	Protein (g)
Macaroni cheese			
per serving:	250	31	18
Cajun chicken fettucine			
for 2:	500	65	40
per serving:	250	33	20
Vegetable curry			
for 2:	400	80	12
per serving:	200	40	6
Char-grilled chicken risotto			
for 2:	365	44	22
per serving:	183	22	11
Chicken linguine with salsa verde			
for 2:	400	56	28
per serving:	200	28	14
Tomato and Mascarpone risotto			
for 2:	365	62	7
per serving:	186	31	4
Tuna and pasta bake			
for 2:	400	48	28
per serving:	200	24	14
Chicken curry			
for 2:	400	88	24
per serving:	200	44	12

Meal	Weight (g)	Carbs (g)	Protein (g)
Chicken fajitas with salsa and sour cream dips			
for 2:	490	80	48
per serving:	245	40	24
Steak fajitas			
for 2:	460	83	41
per serving:	230	42	21
Sweet and sour chicken			
for 2:	300	72	21
per serving:	150	36	11

Indian meals

Unfortunately, different take-away outlets vary in their preparation and content of seemingly identical meals. Some may add sugar to their recipes whereas others may not, so it's probably best to severely restrict Indian take-away meals on this diet – or simply ask whether sugar is added to a selected meal. If so, ask for it to be left out.

This does not, however, mean that Indian food is forbidden. On the contrary, there are other ways of enjoying this delicious food whilst still keeping to a low-GI diet and a hectic lifestyle. Obviously, the simplest way to enjoy the food and be sure of the exact GI value is to cook it yourself. But if you really have virtually no time – or you simply don't want to cook (or can't cook) – there is a perfect fast food alternative: microwavable ready-prepared Indian meals are widely available from supermarkets and are ready in less than five minutes.

However, you must choose carefully because some are low GI and others are very high GI. *Read the label!* The nutritional content of the meal is printed on the packaging and a quick check of the total carbohydrate content of the meal will instantly tell you whether you can include it in your low-GI diet or not.

Incidentally, the external appearance of the packaging will give no indication whatsoever of the contents: the following Indian meals – all from the same outlet – are virtually identical in packaging and size, yet vary from low GI, at 10 grams of carbohydrate, to quite high GI, at 26 grams of carbohydrate per meal. We have even seen a meal in this range at an incredible 77 grams of carbohydrate! So you really must check to find out which to buy and which to leave on the shelf. The protein content as well as the carbohydrate content has been described below for each meal to demonstrate how nutritious they can be.

Indian meals that can be safely included in a low-GI diet

Meal	Weight (g)	Carbs (g)	Protein (g)
Chicken korma	350	13	45
Chicken balti	350	14	38
Chicken makhani	350	24	39
Chicken sag	350	14	39
Chicken tikka masala	350	26	43
Chicken tariwala	350	16	39
Chicken kashmiri	350	24	39
Prawn piri	250	23	18
King prawn makhani	350	10	21
Lamb bhuna	350	21	37
Lamb rogan josh	350	18	45

Chapter 11 Sweet stuff

Pudding can be the healthiest part of any main meal – provided you choose low GI. Substitute the high-GI cakes and pastries with low-GI fruits with cream, or sorbet, crêpes or crème brûlée, and you can literally have your cake and diet!

Lemon syllabub

For 2
75 ml dry white wine
1 tbsp freshly squeezed lemon juice
1 tsp finely grated lemon rind
1½ tbsp caster sugar
150 ml double cream
Fresh mint leaves, to garnish

- *Mix together the white wine, lemon juice, lemon rind and sugar in a medium bowl.*
- *Stir in the cream and spoon into wine glasses.*
- *Chill in the fridge for 2–3 hours and serve, garnished with fresh mint leaves.*

*Carbohydrate content per serving: **15** grams*

Strawberries with blueberry purée

For 2   150 grams blueberries, washed
2 tbsp water
25 grams icing sugar
100 ml double cream
200 grams strawberries, washed and hulled

- Place the blueberries, water and sugar in a medium saucepan and simmer for 4–5 minutes.
- Set aside to cool.
- Strain the blueberries to purée.
- Whip the double cream.
- Arrange the strawberries on dessert plates, top with whipped cream and drizzle the blueberry purée beside the strawberries.
- Serve immediately.

*Carbohydrate content per serving: **30** grams*

Raspberry cream

For 2
1 tbsp caster sugar
4 tbsp cold water
200 grams fresh raspberries, washed
200 ml whipped cream

- *Dissolve the sugar in the water in a small saucepan.*
- *Bring to the boil and simmer until reduced to about half.*
- *Add the raspberries (setting aside 4 raspberries for garnishing) and gently simmer for 5 minutes.*
- *Blend the mixture and set aside to cool.*
- *Fold the raspberry purée into the whipped cream.*
- *Spoon the mixture into dessert dishes.*
- *Garnish with the remaining raspberries.*

*Carbohydrate content per serving: **17** grams*

Strawberries in raspberry cream

For 2
100 grams strawberries, washed and hulled, then halved lengthways
Raspberry cream (above)

- *Stir the strawberries into the raspberry cream and serve immediately.*

*Carbohydrate content per serving: **19** grams*

Crêpes suzette

Crêpes can be made by either the traditional method or by using a commercial crêpe-maker, as described on page 96.

For 2   6 crêpes
5 tbsp freshly squeezed orange juice
2 tbsp freshly squeezed lemon juice
2 tbsp Cointreau
1 tsp caster sugar
25 grams butter

- *Mix together the orange juice, lemon juice, Cointreau and sugar in a medium mixing bowl.*
- *Heat the butter in a medium frying pan and gently heat the sauce mixture.*
- *Lay a crêpe on the citrus mixture in the pan, allow the crêpe to absorb the mixture for about 30 seconds, then fold in half and remove from the pan.*
- *Add each of the other crêpes in a similar manner.*
- *Serve immediately.*

*Carbohydrate content per serving: **30** grams*

Dark chocolate mousse

For 2   45 grams dark chocolate (minimum 70 per cent cocoa
         content)
         20 ml fresh full-cream milk
         50 ml fresh double cream
         4 fresh mint leaves, to garnish

- *Grate about 5 grams (very little) of the chocolate and set aside.*
- *Break up the chocolate into small pieces, place in a heat-safe bowl and set the bowl over a pan of gently simmering hot water. Stir the chocolate from the edges of the bowl as it gradually melts.*
- *Heat the milk, then stir the milk into the chocolate.*
- *Set aside to cool.*
- *Whip the double cream until stiff, then fold the cream into the chocolate mixture.*
- *Transfer the chocolate mousse to ramekin dishes.*
- *Sprinkle a little grated chocolate over each dish, garnish with mint leaves and serve immediately.*

*Carbohydrate content per serving: **10** grams*

Lemon sorbet

For 2
300 ml cold water
75 grams granulated sugar
6 tbsp freshly squeezed lemon juice
1 tbsp grated lemon rind
1 egg white
15 grams caster sugar

- *Pour 100 ml of the water into a medium saucepan and stir in the granulated sugar.*
- *Heat the mixture over a low heat, stirring constantly until the sugar dissolves.*
- *Remove from the heat and strain the mixture.*
- *Stir in the remaining water, lemon juice and lemon rind.*
- *Pour the mixture into a suitable container and chill in the freezer for 20–30 minutes, then stir.*
- *Freeze the lemon mixture for a further 45–60 minutes.*
- *Beat the egg white until stiff and whisk in the caster sugar.*
- *Whisk the lemon mixture and gradually fold in the egg white.*
- *Freeze for 30–40 minutes and whisk again.*
- *Freeze for 2–3 hours, then scoop the lemon sorbet into appropriate dessert dishes and serve immediately.*

*Carbohydrate content per serving: **23** grams*

Red fruit fool

For 2   150 grams mixed fruit: raspberries, redcurrants and
         rhubarb (chopped)
         4 tbsp water
         25 grams caster sugar
         1 tbsp freshly squeezed lemon juice
         150 ml fresh double cream
         4 fresh mint leaves, to garnish

- *Place the mixed fruit, water, sugar and lemon juice in a medium saucepan, bring to the boil, then lower the heat and simmer gently until the fruit softens.*
- *Blend until smooth and set aside to cool.*
- *Whisk the cream until firm and fold into the purée.*
- *Transfer to a medium bowl and chill before serving, garnished with fresh mint leaves.*

*Carbohydrate content per serving: **18** grams*

....

Custard fruit fool

For 2

- *As for red fruit fool (above), substituting cream with custard.*

*Carbohydrate content per serving: **28** grams*

....

Yoghurt fruit fool

For 2

- *As for red fruit fool (above), substituting cream with Greek yoghurt.*

*Carbohydrate content per serving: **23** grams*

Chapter 12 Vinaigrettes, dips, dressings and sauces

French vinaigrette

For 2   4 tbsp extra-virgin olive oil
1 tbsp white wine vinegar
½ tsp mustard powder
½ garlic clove, peeled and chopped finely
Pinch of rock salt
Freshly ground black pepper

- *Add the ingredients of the dressing to a screw-top jar, and shake to mix well.*

Carbohydrate content per serving: negligible

Passata vinaigrette

For 2   3 tbsp extra-virgin olive oil
3 tbsp passata (or tomato juice)
1 tbsp red wine vinegar
½ garlic clove, peeled and grated
Pinch of rock salt
Freshly ground black pepper

- *Add the ingredients of the vinaigrette to a screw-top jar and mix well.*

Carbohydrate content per serving: 3 grams

Oriental vinaigrette

For 2   5 tbsp extra-virgin olive oil
1 tbsp white wine vinegar
1 tbsp light soy sauce
1 tbsp sweet sherry
1 tsp sesame oil
1 slice of fresh ginger root, peeled and chopped finely
Freshly ground black pepper

- *Mix the ingredients in a screw-top jar and shake well.*

*Carbohydrate content per serving: **1** gram*

Honey and orange vinaigrette

For 4   5 tbsp extra-virgin olive oil
1 tbsp white wine vinegar
1 tbsp honey
2 tbsp freshly squeezed orange juice
1 tsp orange zest

- *Mix together the ingredients in a screw-top jar and shake well.*

*Carbohydrate content per serving: **7** grams*

Lemon and coriander vinaigrette

For 2
5 tbsp extra-virgin olive oil
1 tbsp white wine vinegar
1 small garlic clove, peeled and chopped finely
1 tbsp freshly squeezed lemon juice
1 tbsp chopped fresh coriander
Freshly ground black pepper

- *Mix together the ingredients in a screw-top jar and shake thoroughly.*

Carbohydrate content per serving: negligible

....

Balsamic vinaigrette

For 2
4 tbsp extra-virgin olive oil
1 tbsp balsamic vinegar
½ garlic clove, peeled and chopped finely
Pinch of rock salt
Freshly ground black pepper

- *Place all of the ingredients into a screw-top jar and mix thoroughly.*

Carbohydrate content per serving: negligible

Lemon vinaigrette

For 8   250 ml extra-virgin olive oil
60 ml freshly squeezed lemon juice
Freshly ground black pepper

- *Add the ingredients of the vinaigrette to a large screw-top jar and shake vigorously to mix.*

Carbohydrate content per serving: <1 gram

Basil pesto sauce

For 2   40 grams chopped fresh basil leaves
1 garlic clove, peeled and chopped
25 grams pine nuts, lightly toasted
25 grams Parmesan cheese, freshly grated
Small pinch of rock salt
Freshly ground black pepper
40 ml extra-virgin olive oil

- *Add the basil, garlic, pine nuts, cheese and seasoning to a blender, and chop finely.*
- *Continue to blend as the olive oil is gradually added until a smooth, even consistency is obtained.*

*Carbohydrate content per serving: **2** grams*

Chilli and coriander vinaigrette
For 1   1 tsp chopped fresh coriander
¼ green chilli, deseeded and finely diced
2 tbsp French vinaigrette (page 206)

- *Place all of the ingredients into a screw-top jar and mix thoroughly.*

Carbohydrate content per serving: negligible

Mayonnaise
For 6   2 egg yolks from large, free-range eggs
1 garlic clove, peeled and chopped finely
1 tsp Dijon mustard
1 tsp white wine vinegar
200 ml extra-virgin olive oil
Pinch of rock salt
Freshly ground black pepper

- *Place the egg yolks, garlic, mustard and white wine vinegar in a food processor and blend for a few seconds, then – with the motor running – add the olive oil slowly and evenly.*
- *Season to taste, adding a little extra white wine vinegar if necessary.*

Carbohydrate content per serving: negligible

Creamy curry mayonnaise

For 6   1 tbsp extra-virgin olive oil
½ small onion, peeled and diced finely
1 small garlic clove, peeled and chopped finely
1 tbsp medium curry powder
75 ml red wine
1 tbsp sweet sherry
1 tsp freshly squeezed lemon juice
1 bay leaf
Pinch of rock salt
Freshly ground black pepper
200 ml mayonnaise (opposite)
30 ml single cream

- *Heat the extra-virgin olive oil in a medium frying pan and gently sauté the onion and garlic for 2–3 minutes.*
- *Stir in the curry powder and cook for another 2–3 minutes.*
- *Add the wine, sherry, lemon juice and bay leaf, and season to taste.*
- *Bring to the boil, lower the heat and gently simmer for about 8–10 minutes, then remove from the heat and set aside to cool.*
- *When cool, remove the bay leaf and slowly add the sauce to the mayonnaise, stirring constantly.*
- *When fully combined, add the cream slowly, once again stirring constantly.*
- *Cool in the fridge for 2–3 hours before serving.*

*Carbohydrate content per serving: **2** grams*

Coriander pesto sauce

For 2   30 grams fresh coriander leaves
1 garlic clove, peeled and chopped
25 grams pine nuts
25 grams grated Parmesan cheese
Pinch of rock salt
Freshly ground black pepper
40 ml extra-virgin olive oil

- *Add the coriander, garlic, pine nuts, cheese and seasoning to a blender, and chop finely.*
- *Continue to blend as the olive oil is gradually added until a smooth, even consistency is obtained.*

Carbohydrate content per serving: 1 gram

Lemon butter sauce

For 2   50 grams unsalted butter
3 tbsp freshly squeezed lemon juice

- *Melt the butter in a small saucepan, stir in the lemon juice and heat through gently for about a minute.*

Carbohydrate content per serving: 2 grams

Leek and lemon butter sauce

For 4 1 medium leek
100 grams butter
2 tbsp freshly squeezed lemon juice
1 tbsp chopped fresh basil
Freshly ground black pepper

- *Lightly steam the leek, and chop into 1–2 cm segments.*
- *Melt the butter in a medium saucepan, stir in the chopped leek, lemon juice, chopped basil and freshly ground black pepper, and serve immediately.*

*Carbohydrate content per serving: **2** grams*

Tomato and coriander salsa

For 2 4 large plum tomatoes, chopped
3 spring onions, finely chopped
½ small green chilli, deseeded and finely chopped
1 tbsp chopped fresh coriander
Pinch of rock salt
Freshly ground black pepper
French vinaigrette (see page 206)
Sprigs of fresh coriander, to garnish

- *Mix together the tomatoes, onion, chilli and chopped coriander, and season to taste.*
- *Drizzle the vinaigrette over the salsa and garnish with fresh coriander.*

*Carbohydrate content per serving: **7** grams*

Tomato sauce

For 4   400 gram tin peeled plum tomatoes
           1 tbsp tomato purée
           1 tsp granulated sugar
           1 tbsp chopped fresh basil, or 1 tsp dried basil
              (optional)
           Freshly ground black pepper
           Dash of Worcestershire sauce

- *Drain the tomatoes and pour into a small saucepan.*
- *Stir in the tomato purée, sugar and herbs, and season to taste.*
- *Return 1 tablespoon of tomato juice to the pan and bring to a gentle simmer for 5 minutes. Cool the sauce before using.*
- *Add a dash of Worcestershire sauce to the remaining tomato juice and drink – enjoy!*

Carbohydrate content per serving: **6** *grams*

Satay sauce

For 4
1 tbsp extra-virgin olive oil
1 small red onion, peeled and chopped finely
1 garlic clove, peeled and chopped finely
1 small red chilli, deseeded and chopped finely
3 tbsp peanut butter
100 ml coconut cream
½ tsp Worcestershire sauce

- *Heat the extra-virgin olive oil in a small saucepan and sauté the onion, garlic and chilli for 1–2 minutes.*
- *Remove from the heat and stir in the peanut butter, coconut milk and Worcestershire sauce.*
- *Heat through over low heat, then pour into a ramekin dish.*
- *Cover and allow to cool.*

*Carbohydrate content per serving: **9** grams*

Horseradish sauce

For 4
100 ml crème fraîche
1 tbsp grated horseradish
½ tsp caster sugar
2 tsp white wine vinegar
Pinch of rock salt
Freshly ground black pepper

- *Blend the ingredients together, then chill in the fridge for 2–3 hours before use.*

*Carbohydrate content per serving: **2** grams*

Chilli mayonnaise

For 3   1 small red chilli, deseeded and finely chopped
         (replace with a large red chilli if you like it hot!)
         1 garlic clove, peeled and finely chopped
         1 tsp tomato purée
         2–3 drops Tabasco sauce
         100 ml mayonnaise (page 210, or commercial)
         Pinch of rock salt
         Freshly ground black pepper
         Fresh coriander leaves, to garnish

- *Add the ingredients to a food processor and blend until smooth.*
- *Chill for 2–3 hours before serving, garnished with fresh coriander leaves.*

*Carbohydrate content per serving: **1** gram*

Guacamole

For 2
1 large ripe Hass avocado, halved, stoned, peeled and finely diced
½ garlic clove, peeled and finely grated
½ small onion, peeled and finely chopped
½ ripe plum tomato, peeled, deseeded and finely chopped
½ fresh green chilli, deseeded and finely chopped
2 tsp freshly squeezed lime juice
1 tbsp crème fraîche
Freshly ground black pepper

- *Blend together the avocado, garlic, onion, tomato, chilli, lime juice and crème fraîche.*
- *Season to taste and chill before serving.*

*Carbohydrate content per serving: **5** grams*

Tomato salsa

For 2
4 large vine-ripened tomatoes, deseeded and finely chopped
1 medium red onion, peeled and diced
1 garlic clove, peeled and grated
1 green chilli, deseeded and finely chopped
1 tbsp chopped fresh basil
1 tbsp chopped fresh coriander
1 tbsp extra-virgin olive oil

- *Mix together the ingredients in a medium bowl, cover and chill.*

*Carbohydrate content per serving: **8** grams*

Chapter **13** Take the 4-week challenge

On this programme, you will start to lose weight within the first week and you will notice a definite change in your body shape within 2 weeks. So take the 4-week challenge and change your life for ever. This is not an absolutely strict day-by-day programme so you can mix-and-match within the plan. For example, if you don't like eggs, substitute with porridge or yoghurt and fruit. Or exchange a meat dish for vegetarian. The beauty of this diet lies in the immense variety of foods included, but if you do change the plan you must keep your daily intake of carbohydrate to less than 50 grams. On this programme, you really will eat yourself slim and healthy.

Week 1

Sunday
Breakfast: Bacon and eggs
Lunch: Spicy chicken drumsticks
Dinner: Scallops and asparagus with sweet chilli sauce

Monday
Breakfast: Fresh fruit with natural yoghurt
Lunch: Chicken and cashew salad
Dinner: Beef kebabs

Tuesday
Breakfast: Carrot and apple juice
Avocado on toast
Lunch: Prawn mayonnaise open sandwich
Dinner: Vegetable goulash

Wednesday

Breakfast:	Scrambled eggs with tomato
Lunch:	Chilli beef salad
Dinner:	Beefburgers with herbs

Thursday

Breakfast:	Porridge
Lunch:	Salmon with crème fraîche
Dinner:	Spinach and Emmental crêpes

Friday

Breakfast:	Raspberry and orange smoothie
	Breakfast tortilla
Lunch:	Carrot and coriander soup
Dinner:	Chicken chop suey

Saturday

Breakfast:	Mozzarella and tomato omelette
Lunch:	Crab and herb salad
Dinner:	Duck with plum sauce

Week 2

Sunday

Breakfast:	Emmental and prosciutto bagel
Lunch:	Chilli aubergine
Dinner:	Honey-glazed pork

Monday

Breakfast:	Blueberry milkshake
	Continental breakfast: cold meats, sun-dried tomatoes, Emmental cheese and apple
Lunch:	Tomato, ginger and orange salad
Dinner:	Spaghetti Bolognese

Tuesday

Breakfast:	Pancetta and egg crêpes

Lunch: Tuna mayonnaise open sandwich
Dinner: Thai chicken with lemongrass and ginger

Wednesday
Breakfast: Fresh fruit with natural yoghurt
Lunch: Fettuccine with spinach and sage
Dinner: Char-grilled tofu kebabs with satay sauce

Thursday
Breakfast: Raspberry and grapefruit juice
                Porridge
Lunch: Bacon, lettuce and tomato open sandwich
Dinner: Duck with plum sauce

Friday
Breakfast: Char-grilled mushrooms with scrambled eggs
Lunch: Spicy vegetables
Dinner: Milanese risotto

Saturday
Breakfast: Avocado on toast
Lunch: Roast ham with Leerdammer cheese and
                mustard
Dinner: Chicken tikka

Week 3
Sunday
Breakfast: Berry zest juice
                Bacon and eggs
Lunch: Char-grilled pepper salad with herb
                mayonnaise
Dinner: Grilled pepper steak with French beans

Monday
Breakfast: Sun-dried tomatoes and herbs bagel
Lunch: Tomato and basil soup
Dinner: Peperonata

Tuesday
Breakfast: Mushroom and chicken crêpes
Lunch: Prawn mayonnaise open sandwich
Dinner: Basil pesto turkey with char-grilled
               vegetables and sesame seeds

Wednesday
Breakfast: Mango and strawberry milkshake
               Continental breakfast: cold meats, sun-dried
               tomatoes, Emmental cheese and apple
Lunch: Feta and olive salad
Dinner: Spicy turkey kebabs

Thursday
Breakfast: Poached eggs
Lunch: Carrot and coriander soup
Dinner: Nasi Goreng

Friday
Breakfast: Char-grilled mushrooms with scrambled eggs
Lunch: Tuna mayonnaise open sandwich
Dinner: Sweet and sour pork

Saturday
Breakfast: Citrus stinger
               Breakfast tortilla
Lunch: Lemon and chicken soup
Dinner: Lasagne

Week 4
Sunday
Breakfast: Avocado on toast
Lunch: Rocket and olive salad
Dinner: Chicken satay with lime

Monday
Breakfast: Scrambled eggs and asparagus

Lunch: Chicken with mayonnaise and avocado
Dinner: Penne rigate with mixed veg

Tuesday
Breakfast: Continental breakfast: cold meats, sun-dried
                tomatoes, Emmental cheese and apple
Lunch: Gazpacho
Dinner: Spaghetti Bolognese

Wednesday
Breakfast: Porridge
Lunch: Egg mayonnaise sandwich
Dinner: Balti chicken

Thursday
Breakfast: Raspberry and orange smoothie
                Toasted cheese (1 slice)
Lunch: Avocado open sandwich
Dinner: Pork with ginger

Friday
Breakfast: Emmental and prosciutto bagel
Lunch: Tomato and basil soup
Dinner: Coconut okra curry

Saturday
Breakfast: Grilled apples with pineapple and mint
Lunch: Scallop and calamari salad
Dinner: Lemon chicken with cashew nuts

Part III
Health and Exercise

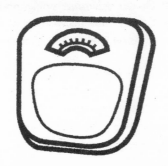

Chapter **14** Low GI for health

You don't need to read this chapter – it simply explains the medical reasons for the diet's success. When you understand how healthy you will become on this diet – as well as slimming easily – you will keep to the lifestyle for ever. Because this is a *lifestyle* – not just a diet.

Insulin

Insulin is a hormone produced by an organ called the pancreas. It has profound effects on every cell in the body. Production of insulin is stimulated by carbohydrates in our diet, and to a much lesser degree by protein. It is not stimulated by fats in the diet. So far, so good. But what is the role of insulin and why is it so bad?

The first point to emphasise is that insulin itself is not bad; in fact, a certain amount of insulin is absolutely essential for health. The problem is that our modern diet makes far too much insulin.

Why is this bad?

Firstly, and most relevant to dieting, insulin causes excess calories to be stored as fat. Even worse, it actually prevents the breakdown of fat. So not only does insulin *make* fat (which you are trying to lose) but it also prevents you burning body fat. Now you can understand why you must reduce insulin to diet successfully.

But too much insulin has other serious effects on health:

- Increased cholesterol levels
- Increased risk of heart disease
- High blood pressure
- Obesity

- Arthritis
- Diabetes
- Kidney failure
- Visual problems

But just when you think the situation cannot get worse, it does! As we make more and more insulin in response to more and more high-GI foods, the cells of the body become less responsive to the hormone. Our body cells become resistant to insulin and the condition of *insulin resistance* develops. And as the cells become more resistant to the effects of the high levels of circulating insulin, the only way that our bodies can compensate is to produce even more! This is the condition called 'hyperinsulinism' – or, more simply, far too much insulin.

As the levels increase, eventually the pancreas cannot make enough insulin for the needs of our body and we develop diabetes, which has to be treated by diet, tablets or even more insulin by injection.

The main complications of diabetes are heart disease, damage to the nervous system, kidney failure and blindness. In fact, diabetes is the commonest cause of blindness in those under 65 in the United Kingdom. And all of these dreadful effects are the direct consequence of a disease which, in many cases, results from a high-GI diet!

Let us summarise the problem:

- Insulin is a hormone which has effects on every cell in the body.
- Insulin is absolutely essential for health but too much can make you ill.
- High-GI foods are the main stimulus for insulin production.
- Too many high-GI foods make too much insulin.

But insulin doesn't just affect diseases such as heart disease and diabetes: it can also be associated with irregular periods and miscarriage. Many women with Polycystic Ovarian Syndrome (PCOS) make too much insulin. This causes:

- Obesity
- Irregular periods
- Skin problems, such as acne
- Abnormal facial hair

By lowering the insulin level in these patients, all of these symptoms improve.

Reduce your insulin levels with a low-GI diet and you will not only regain your bikini shape but be much healthier at the same time!

Insulin levels cannot be lowered by medication. The obvious solution is to reduce its production by following a low-GI diet.

But insulin is not the only factor to be considered. A healthy diet must include all of the essential nutrients – amino acids, essential fatty acids, vitamins and minerals. This low-GI diet has been carefully designed to include all of the essential nutrients, which have been shown to help prevent heart disease, high blood pressure and even some cancers!

Here is a list of the main nutrients essential for health. You don't need to understand this, but just follow this low-GI diet and you will feel healthier within days.

- *Essential amino acids* These are provided by the proteins in animal and plant products: meat, fish, poultry, shellfish, vegetables, fruit, eggs and dairy produce. While plants certainly have proteins, the only plant source with *complete* proteins is soya. By contrast, all animal products have complete proteins, so the easiest way to ensure you have all the amino acids you need is to eat some meat, fish or dairy products.

- *Omega-3 fatty acids* High concentrations in oily fish such as salmon, mackerel, herrings, sardines and tuna, omega-3 fatty acids can also be obtained from egg yolks, as well as nuts and certain seeds (e.g. flaxseed oil).

- *Omega-6 fatty acids* In egg yolks, seeds (particularly sunflower, safflower and sesame), whole grains and some vegetables.

- *Vitamin A* Typical foods with high concentrations of vitamin A are fish, egg yolk, butter, cheese, carrots, red peppers, spinach, tomatoes and mangetout.

- *Vitamin B_1 (thiamin)* Excellent sources of B_1 are pork, fresh fish (especially salmon), certain nuts (cashews, brazils, peanuts, pine nuts) and sesame seeds.

- *Vitamin B_2 (riboflavin)* In dairy products (cream and cheese), liver, beef, chicken, eggs, fish, shellfish, mushrooms, avocado and almonds.

- *Vitamin B_3 (niacin)* High concentrations are found in fish (especially salmon and tuna), meat, chicken, liver and eggs.

- *Vitamin B_6 (pyridoxine)* In fish (especially tuna), meat (particularly pork), liver, chicken, avocados, nuts (especially walnuts and cashews), tomatoes and tomato purée.

- *Vitamin B_{12} (cyanocobalamin)* This is the only vitamin not found in plants. It is present in highest concentrations in liver, seafood, fish (especially sardines, salmon and tuna) and eggs, and in lesser amounts in milk products and meats. Vegetarians are therefore recommended to take a vitamin supplement to obtain B_{12}.

- *Folate* The highest concentration of folate occurs in liver, but there are also good concentrations in most vegetables (especially green vegetables), meat, poultry, fish, shellfish, eggs and nuts (particularly peanuts and cashews).

- *Vitamin C* Apart from liver and kidney, vitamin C is not present in animal foods and has to be obtained from vegetables (especially red and green peppers, mangetout, tomato and broccoli) and fruit (strawberries and citrus fruits).

- *Vitamin D* This is where oily fish are in a class of their own, providing by far the highest levels of vitamin D compared with any other food group; mackerel, herring, salmon and tuna are particularly rich sources of this vitamin. There is a small amount of vitamin D in eggs and butter.

- *Vitamin E* The dietary requirements for this vitamin are provided in the diet by nuts (almonds, hazelnuts, peanuts), olives, tomato purée, avocado and fish.

- *Vitamin K* The best dietary source is undoubtedly green vegetables, such as broccoli, cabbage, lettuce, spring onions and spinach.

- *Selenium* This essential mineral is present in onions, tomatoes, broccoli, beansprouts and fish.

- *Iron* You will obtain sufficient amounts of this important mineral from fish, nuts, liver, meat, chicken, sesame seeds and green vegetables.

- *Manganese* In eggs, nuts and green vegetables.

- *Copper* Nuts, mushrooms and green vegetables are all good sources of copper.

- *Zinc* Excellent sources include eggs, sesame seeds, nuts (especially cashew nuts and almonds), herbs and many vegetables.

- *Potassium* This is abundant in fish, herbs, garlic, onion, vegetables, mushrooms and citrus fruit.
- *Calcium* Important for the manufacture of bones, this is found in dairy products, fish, green vegetables (especially broccoli and parsley) and herbs.
- *Sulphur* You can obtain this from garlic, onions, fish, eggs, nuts, cabbage and meat.

The recipes have been carefully devised to ensure a nutritionally balanced diet; for more ideas on how to balance your meals, turn to the menu plans on pages 218–22.

What happens if you break your diet occasionally?

Unfortunately, this diet is not as forgiving as some others. In a calorie-controlled diet, you can eat some chocolate cake and make up for the extra calories by eating very little for the rest of the day – but low-calorie diets mess up the body's chemical balance and don't work.

In a low-GI diet, if you consume more than 50 grams of carbohydrate per day, your body will respond by depositing the excess calories as fat. So you can't have many lapses, or it simply won't work. A biscuit here and a pastry there and it will all go to fat.

Of course, nobody's perfect, and no one can stick to all the rules all the time. The occasional lapse with a sandwich or an extra piece of fruit will merely cause the diet to fail on that day only. So don't panic if you break your diet occasionally, it's only human.

By satisfying your natural hunger in a natural way, for the first time you have a diet that is working with you, not against you. Remember, within a few days of commencing the diet your body will automatically readjust, and you will no longer need sugars; the addiction will disappear. Your body will be on automatic pilot! And you will not be hungry during the early phase of the diet, the most difficult period in most diets.

And now to the good part!

After a few weeks on the diet, your body automatically adjusts to the new insulin levels. This means that you will almost certainly be able to eat more than 50 grams of carbohydrate per day after the weight-loss phase of the diet and still not gain weight. Obviously you can't eat too much or your weight will increase, but you will be able to 'mini-binge' safely on occasions.

This diet works – and it lasts!

Chapter 15 Shape up for summer

You don't have to exercise to diet successfully and lose weight, but you do have to exercise if you want to be really healthy. Why? Because even a little exercise improves the circulation, which is the basis for good health.

Moderate exercise does not involve jogging, gym training, aerobics or any of the other popular exercise regimes that come and go without seeming to make any significant impact. The reason these exercise programmes are only successful for the fortunate few is that they are really not practical and unless you are totally committed to an exercise regime of this nature you will give up after a short time.

Severe exercise is seldom successful as part of a weight-loss programme because it doesn't make sense medically. When you exercise strenuously you become very hungry. Unless you have an iron will, you must inevitably eat – usually much more than the calories you have used up in exercise. And exercise stimulates insulin, which makes more body fat! Jogging causes stress to knees and ankles – usually on knees and ankles which have had very little exercise for many years!

Weight training in the gym and aerobics are similarly non-sensical exercises for overweight people. When you haven't exercised for years you are quite simply 'out of condition'. What exactly does this mean? Your muscles have wasted so you tire easily, your breathing can't cope with excessive exertion and your cardiovascular function (heart and circulation) cannot increase sufficiently to compensate for the massive demands suddenly being placed on the muscles which require oxygen during exercise – fast! The result for the out-of-condition, overweight individual, who embarks upon such a sudden crash programme to lose weight as quickly as possible by unaccustomed exercise, is at best physical exhaustion and pain and at worst a heart attack!

Incidentally, pain during exercise is a danger signal. It is a warning that there is a build-up of lactic acid in the muscles which is the body's method of warning you that the muscles are not obtaining sufficient oxygen. If you continue to try to break through the pain barrier you are increasingly likely to place your life in danger. The maxim 'no pain, no gain' is dangerous.

The best exercise for unfit people is walking. Yes, it is as simple as that! Walking 15–20 minutes per day is medically proven to significantly improve fitness levels. Why? Because walking increases the blood flow to the muscles, improving circulation and heart function. And moderate walking each day has no dangerous or detrimental effects on health. So the single most important exercise for anyone unfit and on a diet is moderate walking – about 20 minutes per day. But this does not mean that you have to walk in the morning (before work) or in the evening (after work). The easiest way to exercise is to include it in your working day.

Park the car, or get off the bus, 10 minutes' walk from work and you have automatically completed your daily exercise programme. Or walk to lunch 10 minutes from the office.

But walking is not the only part of your daily exercise programme that can be easily included in your working day. The important point is to use the free moments in your day – every day – to maximum effect.

You may not think that you have any free time during the day, but you do! For a moment, just consider how much time you spend sitting at your desk, or even waiting for a meal to cook in the kitchen! All this time, which would otherwise be completely wasted, can be effectively used to exercise, because this is a practical programme designed to fit around your lifestyle – not the other way around. And because the exercise programme fits your lifestyle (as with the diet) it is easy to perform on a regular basis and is therefore bound to be successful.

This exercise programme is quite different from others as it does not involve any movement or any special equipment whatsoever, so it can be performed almost anywhere. How can you possibly exercise without moving? Quite simply, because you contract your muscles against an immovable object, such as a table. Let us provide a simple example. Sit on a dining chair at a normal table, extend your arms in front of you and place your hands palm downwards on the table.

Take a deep breath and, sitting perfectly still, press your hands down on the table surface and keep pressing constantly for 6–8 seconds, then relax. This is a strengthening exercise for the upper back muscles and you will have felt the muscle tension in your upper back during the exercise. Performing this simple exercise 4–5 days per week will result in considerable strengthening of the upper back muscles. And, as you can see, this can be easily performed at home or in the office.

Now that you can appreciate how simply and easily an effective exercise programme can be included in your daily life, we shall describe exercises which can be adapted to virtually every busy lifestyle.

How to exercise – without really trying

So here it is: the 5-minute-a-day exercise plan for everyone who 'doesn't have time to exercise'. Just to make it absolutely impossible for there to be any excuse not to incorporate this into your daily routine, we have adapted exercises that can be done at home, in the office or even in the car! Follow the plan and you will tone up those muscles as the fat disappears.

Always complete the routine in the following sequence:
- Neck exercises
- Improve your bust
- Upper back exercise
- Smooth those arms
- Hips, bums and tums

Neck exercises

Always start your exercise programme with neck exercises. These are almost always forgotten during a typical exercise regime but they are very important because they tone the neck muscles to give a smooth, attractive neck contour.

Warning: Do not perform neck exercises if you have any medical history of neck injury or problems, or if you have any evidence of reduced circulation to the brain. Always consult your doctor before commencing any form of exercise regime.

There are four basic movements required to exercise the full range of movement of the neck.

1. Bend your head forward until your chin touches your chest then lift your head backwards as far as you can. Don't force the movement. You may find that your neck movements are quite stiff, especially if you have not performed neck exercises for many years (or perhaps never!). The flexion of neck movements will gradually increase over a period of a few weeks with regular exercise. Repeat the movement 5 times.

2. Whilst looking straight ahead, bend your neck to the left side and try to place your left ear on your left shoulder. Don't force the movement. Then lift your head to the upright position and try to place your right ear on your right shoulder. Repeat the movement 5 times.

3. With your head in the upright position, turn your head to the right as far as you are able to comfortably achieve, then turn your head in the opposite direction to the left. Repeat the movement 5 times.

4. Tilt your head backwards until the back of your head touches your upper back then rotate your head around to the left until your chin touches your chest. Continue the movement to the right until you have completed a complete rotation of the neck and the back of your head is again resting on the back of your neck. Repeat the movement 5 times.

Perform the opposite rotation by tilting your head backwards until the back of your head touches your upper back, then rotate your head to the right until you complete a rotation. Once again, repeat the exercise 5 times.

Improve your bust

Improving the tone of your chest muscles is very important. By firming these you can increase your bust size without unsightly muscle contours. Exercises for the chest muscles can be performed almost anywhere: in the office or at home – even in the car!

In the office/at home

Clasp both hands together in front of your chest with elbows bent. Take a deep breath in and hold, then press both palms together as firmly as you can; hold the contraction for 6–8 seconds whilst holding your breath, and relax.

In the car

This exercise can only be performed whilst sitting in the car, when the car is not moving and the engine is switched off! Sit upright in the driving seat, extend your arms to the front, place both hands on the outer edges of the steering wheel and grasp the wheel tightly. Take a deep breath in and hold, then press both hands together as firmly as you can, hold the contraction for 6–8 seconds and relax.

Upper back exercise

If you want the 'hour-glass' bikini shape you have to exercise the upper back muscles. There are two simple exercises for the upper back muscles. Once again, we will describe two of the commonest situations: in the office (or at home) and in the car.

In the office/at home

Sit upright in a straight-backed chair, place both hands behind your back and grasp the outer edges of the chair firmly. Take a deep breath in and hold then press both hands together as firmly as you can. Hold the contraction for 6–8 seconds and relax. The second exercise for the muscles of the upper back is described below.

In the car

Once again, it is important to emphasise that these exercises can only be performed when the car is stationary and the engine is switched off – not while driving! Sit upright in the driving seat, extend your arms to the front and place both hands on the outer edges of the steering wheel and grasp the wheel tightly. Take a deep breath in and hold, then try to pull your hands away from one another in an outwards direction, hold the contraction for 6–8 seconds and relax.

The second movement exercises the broad upper back muscles. Sitting upright in the driving seat, extend your arms to the front, place both hands on the lower margin of the steering wheel and grasp the wheel tightly. Take a deep breath in and hold, then try to push your hands downwards towards the floor, hold the contraction for 6–8 seconds and relax.

Smooth those arms

Toning of the upper arm muscles is essential to get rid of the horrible 'dimpled' skin of cellulite.

When a woman increases the tone of her arm muscles, the overlying fat layer gives a smooth contour to the upper arm, which produces an attractive appearance, taking away the undesirable 'bumpy' cellulite.

We begin by increasing the tone of the muscles on the front of the arm. Put your hands by your sides. Bend your left arm up to form a right angle, keeping your elbow level with your waist. Your arm should be in a similar position to when you shake someone's hand. Place your right hand over your left wrist and grasp it. Take a deep breath in and hold. Press up with your left arm while pressing down with your right hand. The left arm should not move during the exercise. Hold the tension for 8–10 seconds, and relax.

Repeat the movement on the right side to exercise the right arm, once again keeping your right elbow level with your waist.

Obviously, having exercised the muscles on the front of the arm (which bend it), we have to exercise the muscles on the back of the arm (which straighten it).

Once again, bend your left arm to a right angle, but this time place your right hand under your left wrist, before grasping it. Take a deep breath in and hold. Press down with your left arm whilst pushing up with your right arm. Hold the tension for 8–10 seconds, and relax.

Repeat the movement on the right side. Hold the tension for 8–10 seconds, and then relax.

Hips, bums and tums

Hips and bums

Toning the leg muscles is easy but you have to be careful! You may be exercising muscles that have not been exercised for years so only do as much exercise as you can safely achieve and no more!

Lie flat on your back. Keeping your leg straight, slowly raise your right leg about 8–10cm off the ground. Hold in this position for 8–10 seconds, then slowly lower your leg to the ground.

Repeat this exercise for the left leg.

Firm that bum

Lie flat on your front. Once again, keeping your leg straight, slowly raise your right leg about 8–10cm off the ground. Hold in this position for 8–10 seconds, then slowly lower your leg to the ground.

Repeat this exercise for the left leg.

Flatten that tum

Like back exercises, this one can cause injuries, because people tend to attack it far too enthusiastically. Only perform the exercise to the level you are able, and that means if you can't do it at this stage, don't!

These are exercises that you may not be accustomed to, and it's not likely that you will be able to perform them easily. You will look better with a slimmer waist from the diet, and as the fat decreases you will gradually be able to perform the abdominal exercise with ease. Do what you can, no more, and never be afraid to stop. No pain, no gain is for fools!

Lie flat on your back with your hands by your sides. Take a deep breath and hold, then gently lift the upper part of your body

Cellulite-busting tips

- Drink at least 1 litre of water per day to re-hydrate
- Cut out the refined carbs
- Increase fruit and veggies in your diet
- More dietary fibre
- Keep alcohol intake low
- Stop smoking
- No junk food
- No fizzy drinks
- Dry body brushing (brush your body all over with a dry brush) and gentle massage will improve the circulation and lymph drainage, helping to remove the accumulated fluids from the cellulite

But the simplest and most effective advice is:
- Follow the Gi Bikini Diet exercise programme at least four times every week
- Walk for 20 minutes every day
- Follow the Gi Bikini Diet!

about 10 cm off the ground (using your abdominal muscles; don't push up with your hands) and hold for 8–10 seconds (or less), then relax. This is all you need to do to tighten your abdominal muscles and improve abdominal shape, but it is a hard exercise in the beginning, so don't over-exert yourself.

On the beach

No, we're not suggesting you work out in the *conventional* sense when you're enjoying your beach holiday, but there are some easy tricks to keep you in shape even on the beach:

- Always choose the sun-lounger furthest from the bar! That way, you will always be sure of some exercise.
- Swim at least 20 minutes per day.
- Take a brisk 20-minute walk along the beach every morning – before the sun is too hot.
- Take the stairs rather than the elevator.
- Check out the fitness programme in your hotel complex.

And that's all you need for a very effective exercise programme to tone your muscles whilst losing weight. Five minutes per day is all it takes. Add 20 minutes' walking three times a week and the programme is complete. The cellulite will be replaced by toned, attractive curves.

Chapter **16** Going on holiday

Now that you have your bikini body you have to make the most of your new figure by choosing the right bikini for your shape. The wrong swimsuit can literally undo all of your hard work because different shapes and fabrics can either make your figure look better – or worse! Select your shape from the list below and choose the swimsuit to match.

Petite figure Pretty, single-colour swimsuit, bikini-style, with subtle trim. Simple ruching at bustline to emphasise curves. If you need to enhance your bustline, padded and push-up styles will do the trick.

Tall and slim You definitely want to show off those legs, so wear bold prints with side-ties or high-cut legs.

Short legs High-cut swimsuits or bikini briefs with side-ties will create the illusion of longer, slimmer legs.

Big bust Plunge neckline swimsuit with underwired bra for extra support. Adjustable shoulder straps are a must.

Firm that bum If you haven't had time to firm your bottom with the exercise programme, go for a one-piece swimsuit, low-cut with extra Lycra for more firming. Choose shorts-style briefs for a bikini.

Flatten that tum Never stripes or plain styles! Bold patterns with firming side panels will smooth out the problem areas.

Pear-shaped Simplicity is the answer. A halter-neck all-in-one with detailed bust-line and plain colours on the lower half. A colourful, sexy sarong completes the picture.

Finally, having worked so hard to get your bikini figure and chosen the perfect bikini, don't let the sun spoil your holiday. Of course, you want a great tan, but be careful – too much sun too quickly is dangerous! Apart from painful sunburn, ultraviolet rays cause skin cancer. Here are some tips to help you make sure you get the best tan *safely*:

- Always apply 30+ sunscreen *before* going outside
- Gradually build up exposure to direct sunlight – no more than 30 minutes' sunbathing per day for the first week
- At all other times, wear a broad-brim hat
- Polarising sunglasses are essential – especially wrap-around models
- Remember the 30-minute rule: at all other times, wear a loose wrap or beach shirt
- Keep hydrated. Drink at least a glass of water every hour
- Don't be fooled by a cool breeze on the beach. The sun is just as hot and the UV rays just as dangerous
- If you're drinking alcohol, have a full glass of water between alcoholic drinks as alcohol can dehydrate you even more
- Always re-apply sunscreen all over as soon as you leave either the pool or the sea after swimming
- *Never* sunbathe between 10am and 2pm
- Even safer, and more effective, is fake tan!

Appendix: The Gi Bikini Diet counter

In general, the following is a simple guide to foods *included* or *excluded* from the diet:

Foods included virtually without restriction
- Fish and shellfish
- Herbs and spices
- Meat and poultry
- Oils and dressings
- Vegetables (except those with a high-carbohydrate content, such as potatoes and parsnips)
- Low-calorie soft drinks
- Tea
- Artificial sweeteners

Foods for which some restrictions apply
- Dairy products
- Drinks (fizzy soft drinks and fruit juices)
- Eggs (up to 7 per week)
- Most fruit (except bananas, mangoes and pineapple)
- Nuts
- Sauces, mustards and stock
- Soups
- Pasta
- Rice
- Bread, flour, grains and cereals
- Pulses
- Cheese – up to 50 g per day
- Alcoholic spirits (whisky, gin, brandy) – maximum of 2 measures per day
- Red wine – maximum of 2 glasses per day
- Dry white wine – maximum of 2 glasses per day

Foods excluded during the initial phase

- Biscuits, cakes and pastries
- Desserts and sugars
- Fast food
- Snack foods
- Chocolate and sweets
- Potatoes and parsnips
- Bananas, mangoes and pineapple
- Jasmine rice
- Beer, lager, cider, sweet white wine, champagne, sherry and port

Whilst the Glycaemic Index is not exactly the same as the carb content, this gives the easiest measure for quick comparisons. In general, high carb equals high GI.

Low-GI foods

Food Item	Carbohydrate (g)	Calories	Food Item	Carbohydrate (g)	Calories
DAIRY PRODUCTS			Stilton	<1	92
BUTTER AND MARGARINE (15 g)			Wensleydale	<1	92
Standard	0	150			
Ghee (clarified)	0	150	**PREPARED CHEESES (25 g)**		
Margarine	<1	110	Cheese strings	<1	82
			(per stick: 21 g)	<1	69
CHEESE (25 g)					
Brie	<1	91	**CREAM (100 ml)**		
Camembert	<1	77	Crème fraiche	3	380
Cheddar	<1	100	Double cream	3	460
Cheshire	<1	95	Single cream	3	330
Cottage	<1	25	Soured cream	4	200
Cream cheese	<1	84			
Edam	<1	88	**MILK (100 ml)**		
Emmental	<1	95	Cow's		
Feta	<1	70	evaporated	11	160
Gloucester	<1	100	full-cream	5	66
Goat's cheese	<1	50	high-calcium	5	49
Halloumi	<1	60	semi-skimmed	5	50
Lancashire	<1	90	skimmed	5	35
Leicester	<1	100	UHT longlife	5	68
Mozzarella	<1	75	Goat's milk	4	60
Parmesan	<1	110	Soya	1	32
Philadelphia cream cheese	2	70			
Ricotta	<1	40			

Food Item	Carbohydrate (g)	Calories
DRINKS		
Coffee (200 ml; decaf)	<1	0
Diet soft drinks (100 ml)		
cola	<1	1
lemonade	<1	3
orange	<1	1
tonic	<1	1
Fruit Shoot (100 ml)		
Orange and peach	<1	5
Light low-sugar orange juice	1	8
Spirits (25 ml)		
Bacardi	<1	53
brandy	<1	53
gin	<1	53
rum	<1	53
vodka	<1	53
whisky	<1	53
Tea		
China	<1	0
Sri Lanka	<1	0
Wine (100 ml)		
red	<1	71
white, dry	<1	75
white, medium	3	77
Sherry (50 ml), dry	2	115
Vermouth (50 ml), dry	2	53
Water		
carbonated	0	0
flavoured (orange and mango)	0	<1
still	0	0
EGGS		
Boiled egg	0	147
Duck's egg (large)	0	160
Fried egg	0	147
Omelette	0	147
Poached egg	0	147
Scrambled egg	0	147
Quail's egg	0	15
FISH AND SHELLFISH		
FISH		
Anchovies (25 g)	<1	45
Bass	<1	90
Bream	<1	135
Calamari	<1	70
Cod	<1	80
Dover sole	<1	80
Haddock		
fresh	<1	100
smoked	<1	100
Herring	<1	230
Kipper	<1	205
Lemon sole	<1	95

Food Item	Carbohydrate (g)	Calories
Mackerel		
peppered	<1	355
smoked	<1	190
Salmon		
fresh	<1	200
tinned	<1	150
smoked	<1	180
Sardines		
fresh	<1	65
tinned (in oil)	<1	220
Swordfish	<1	120
Trout		
rainbow	<1	125
smoked	<1	135
Tuna		
fresh	<1	120
tinned (oil)	<1	180
tinned (brine)	<1	105
Whiting	<1	90
PREPARED FISH PRODUCTS		
Cod fillets	<1	76
Fish fingers (100 g)	13	170
(each)	4	50
SHELLFISH		
Crab		
fresh	<1	120
tinned	1	80
Lobster	<1	120
Mussels	<1	88
Oysters	<1	120
Prawns	<1	100
Scallops	<1	100
HERBS AND SPICES		
FRESH HERBS (1 tbsp)		
All varieties, including basil, coriander, dill, lemon grass, mint, oregano, parsley, rosemary and thyme	<1	15–20
Garlic (1 clove)	<1	3
Horseradish	<1	15–20
Rocket (100 g)	2	15
Watercress	2	15–20
DRIED SPICES (1 tsp)		
All varieties, including allspice, bay leaf, chilli powder, cinnamon, cloves, cumin, fennel, nutmeg, paprika, pepper, salt and turmeric <1		10
Capers	<1	3
Ginger	7	40

Food Item	Carbohydrate (g)	Calories
MEAT		
BEEF		
Beefburgers		
home-made (100 g)	0	180
Fillet steak (100 g)		
trimmed	0	190
untrimmed	0	210
Kidney (100 g)	0	150
Liver (100 g)	0	200
Mince, lean (100 g)	0	124
Round steak (100 g)		
trimmed	0	180
untrimmed	0	200
Rump steak (100 g)		
trimmed	0	190
untrimmed	0	270
Sirloin steak (100 g)		
trimmed	0	170
untrimmed	0	270
T-bone steak (100 g)		
trimmed	0	140
untrimmed	0	170
Topside steak (100 g)		
trimmed	0	150
untrimmed	0	170
LAMB, NATURAL		
Cutlet (40 g)		
trimmed	0	90
untrimmed	0	130
Kidney	0	210
Leg (100 g)		
trimmed	0	200
untrimmed	0	220
Liver (100 g)	4	230
Loin chop (50 g)		
trimmed	0	85
untrimmed	0	180
Shank (100 g)		
trimmed	0	140
untrimmed	0	220
Shoulder (100 g)		
trimmed	0	140
untrimmed	0	260
PORK, NATURAL		
Bacon (100 g)	0	260
Fillet (100 g)	0	170
Leg (100 g)		
trimmed	0	170
untrimmed	0	330
Loin chop (100 g)		
trimmed	0	170
untrimmed	0	350
Medallion (100 g)		
trimmed	0	190
untrimmed	0	300

Food Item	Carbohydrate (g)	Calories
Mince, lean (100 g)	0	80
Spare ribs (100 g)	0	110
Steak (100 g)		
trimmed	0	160
untrimmed	0	260
PORK, PREPARED		
Gammon steak (100 g)	0	160
Ham (100 g)		
trimmed	0	100
untrimmed	0	140
wafer thin	<1	105
OILS, MAYONNAISE AND DRESSINGS		
OILS		
Corn oil	0	829
Extra-virgin olive oil	0	823
Virgin olive oil	0	822
Olive oil	0	822
Grapeseed oil	0	829
Groundnut oil	0	829
Peanut oil	0	899
Sesame oil	0	821
Soya oil	0	899
Sunflower oil	0	828
MAYONNAISE AND VINAIGRETTES		
Mayonnaise	1	722
Vinaigrette, home-made	<1	60
Commercial dressings		
French	15	297
low-fat French	9	39
Italian	6	120
low-fat Italian	7	32
VINEGAR (per 15 ml)		
Balsamic	12	10
Cider	<1	2
Red wine	2	5
Rice	<1	5
White wine	0	5
POULTRY		
CHICKEN, NATURAL (100 g)		
Breast		
skinless	0	170
with skin	0	210
Drumstick		
skinless	0	90
with skin	0	110
Thigh		
skinless	0	60
with skin	0	70
Wing		
skinless	0	70

Food Item	Carbohydrate (g)	Calories
with skin	0	90
CHICKEN, PREPARED (100 g)		
Breast roll	0	120
Drumsticks	0	180
Wings, in barbecue marinade	3	232
DUCK (100 g)		
Roast duck		
skinless	0	180
with skin	0	300
TURKEY, NATURAL (100 g)		
Breast		
skinless	0	105
Mince	0	176
TURKEY, PREPARED (100 g)		
Breast roll	4	92

VEGETABLES AND VEGETABLE PRODUCTS

Food Item	Carbohydrate (g)	Calories
Alfalfa sprouts	4	30
Artichoke		
globe	1	8
Jerusalem	9	40
Asparagus	1	12
Aubergine	2	14
Beans		
French	4	25
green	4	25
Beetroot	8	35
Broccoli	1	25
Brussels sprouts	2	25
Cabbage		
bok choy	<1	12
Chinese	<1	8
red	2	22
savoy	2	20
Carrots	8	37
Cauliflower	2	20
Celeriac	5	30
Celery	3	12
Chilli		
green	1	20
red	4	26
Courgettes		
green	2	15
yellow	2	15
Cucumber		
English	6	9
Lebanese	3	12
Fennel	4	12
Herb salad, commercial	2	15
Leek		
standard	3	20

Food Item	Carbohydrate (g)	Calories
baby	3	23
Lettuce		
cos	2	20
curly endive	2	20
iceberg	2	20
radicchio	2	20
Swiss chard	2	20
Mangetout	5	60
Marrow	4	20
Mushrooms		
button	2	25
oyster	5	35
Onion		
brown	4	25
red	4	25
white	4	25
Peas		
fresh green	6	60
tinned	9	67
sugarsnap	5	33
Peppers		
green	3	15
red	4	25
Radish	2	3
Salad leaves, commercial	2	25
Seaweed	<1	10
Spinach	2	30
Spring onion	4	25
Swede	2	10
Tomato		
beefsteak	3	20
cherry	3	20
plum	3	20
plum, tinned/peeled	4	24
round	3	20
vine-ripened	3	20
Turnip	2	12

COMMERCIALLY PREPARED VEGETABLES

Food Item	Carbohydrate (g)	Calories
Sausages, vegetarian		
organic leek and cheese		
(100 g)	11	195
(per sausage)	5	81
Vegetarian quarter-pounder		
burgers	7	164

Medium-GI foods

BREAD, FLOUR AND GRAINS
BREAD

	Carbohydrate (g)	Calories
Bap	30–41	175–246
Bagel	30	140

Food Item	Carbohydrate (g)	Calories
Baguette	23	130
Bran loaf	35	130
Brown bread	11–20	53–97
Croissant	22	207
Focaccia	30	140
Fruit bread	15	77
Hamburger roll	40	215
Naan	50	340
Pitta	12–50	55–230
Roll	25–33	150–270
Tortilla	12–25	67–144
White bread	11–20	50–110
Wholemeal bread	15–20	77–102
FLOUR (per 100 g)		
Corn	90	350
Rice	80	360
Soya		
(full fat)	23	450
(low fat)	28	350
Wheat		
plain/white	77	340
self-raising/white	76	330
wholemeal	65	320
GRAINS (per 100 g)		
Barley		
pearl	84	360
wholegrain	65	300
Bulgar	70	330
Couscous	72	355
Oatmeal	70	400
Wheat germ	45	300
DIPS (100 g)		
Chilli cheese	9	550
Garlic and herb	7	370
Hot salsa	9	40
Hummus	12	190
DAIRY PRODUCTS		
YOGHURT (100 ml)		
Acidophilus	8	25
Blackcurrant	17	141
Blackberry and raspberry	15	125
Creamy bio yoghurt	11	130
Strawberry bio yoghurt	9	114
Vanilla flavour with chocolate rice	19	120
Natural yoghurt		
full-fat	6	120
Greek	8	100
skimmed-milk	6	50

Food Item	Carbohydrate (g)	Calories
DRINKS		
Carbonated soft drinks (150 ml)		
cola	16	60
lemonade	16	62
lemon and lime	16	62
Coffee, caffeinated (200 ml)		
black	<1	<1
cappuccino	10	134
white	3	25
Fruit juice (100 ml)		
grapefruit (unsweetened)	8	35
'traditional'-style lemonade	18	74
orange, fresh	8	33
commercial (unsweetened)	9	37
Wine (100 ml)		
rosé	3	75
white, sweet	6	99
FRUIT		
Apple	10	40
Apricot	7	9
Avocado	2	190
Blackberries (100 g)	12	50
Blueberries (100 g)	13	52
Cherries (100 g)	12	52
Grapefruit	10	51
Grapes (100 g)		
black	15	62
green	12	55
Kiwi fruit	7	35
Lemon	3	11
Lime	<1	8
Melon		
honeydew (100 g)	6	30
rock (100 g)	5	22
water (100 g)	5	22
Nectarine	7	32
Orange	10	42
Passion fruit	3	20
Peach	8	33
Pear	16	64
Pineapple (100 g)	8	37
Plum	8	34
Raspberries (100 g)	5	24
Rhubarb (100 g)	1	8
Strawberries (100 g)	6	28
Tangerine	7	33
Nuts		
Almond	7	610
Brazil	3	680
Hazelnut	6	650
Macadamia	5	740
Peanut	12	560
Pecan	6	690

Food Item	Carbohydrate (g)	Calories
Pine nut	4	690
Pistachio	8	600
Walnut	3	690

PULSES
BEANS

Food Item	Carbohydrate (g)	Calories
Baked beans in tomato sauce	14	75
Black-eye	20	110
Broad	6	150
Butter	12	80
Chickpeas	15	110
Chilli	12	70
Haricot	16	100
Kidney (red)	16	100
Lentils	16	100
Soya		
bean	5	140
tofu	1	75

SAUCES AND MUSTARDS

Food Item	Carbohydrate (g)	Calories
Gravy		
commercial	10	130
powder	5	25
Pasta sauces, commercial		
Bolognese	9	52
pesto	60	550
Salsa, fresh	8	47
Soy	8	40
Sweet and sour	25	100
Tartare	14	263
Tomato	35	155
Tomato ketchup	25	107
White sauce, home-made	20	200
Worcestershire	25	110

MUSTARD

Food Item	Carbohydrate (g)	Calories
English	19	190
French	4	104
Wholegrain	4	140

SOUPS (COMMERCIAL)

Food Item	Carbohydrate (g)	Calories
Chicken noodle (100 ml)	5	27
(per serving)	10	54
Cream of chicken (100 ml)	5	51
(per serving)	10	102
Cream of tomato (100 ml)	11	71
(per serving)	22	142
Cream of mushroom (100 ml)	5	51
(per serving)	10	102
French onion (100 ml)	5	25
(per serving)	10	50
Lentil (100 ml)	8	41
(per serving)	16	82
Minestrone (100 ml)	5	30
(per serving)	10	60
Mulligatawny (100 ml)	7	60
(per serving)	14	120
Vegetable (100 ml)	8	47
(per serving)	16	94

High-GI foods
BISCUITS, CAKES, PASTRIES AND BUNS (100 g)
SWEET BISCUITS

Food Item	Carbohydrate (g)	Calories
Bourbon	70	500
(per biscuit)	8	60
Chocolate chip	70	500
(per biscuit)	7	50
Cream	70	450
(per biscuit)	7	45
Crunch cream	64	520
(per biscuit)	9	75
Custard cream	65	500
(per biscuit)	8	65
Digestive		
chocolate	70	500
(per biscuit)	10	75
plain	65	450
(per biscuit)	10	70
Flapjack	57	475
(per biscuit)	13	110
Ginger	80	450
(per biscuit)	8	45
Jaffa cake	70	370
(per biscuit)	10	20
Kit Kat	60	506
(per biscuit)	12	106
Kit Kat Orange	60	506
(per biscuit)	12	106
Rich Tea style	75	460
(per biscuit)	6	35
Shortbread		
round	65	500
(per slice)	10	80
Scotch finger	70	510
(per piece)	11	90
Shortcake	60	500
(per biscuit)	6	90
Wagon Wheel	68	425
(per biscuit)	27	170

CRACKERS AND CRISPBREADS

Food Item	Carbohydrate (g)	Calories
Cream cracker	65	450
(per cracker)	5	30
Oatcakes	65	450
(per biscuit)	6	45

Food Item	Carbohydrate (g)	Calories	Food Item	Carbohydrate (g)	Calories
Rye crispbread	70	330	Viennese cakes	60	500
(per crispbread)	6	25	(per cake: 50 g)	30	250
Water biscuit	80	450			
(per biscuit)	5	30	**PASTRIES**		
Wholemeal cracker	75	420	Croissant	40	350
(per cracker)	5	30	(per croissant)	25	210
			Danish		
CAKES AND BUNS			apple	45	300
Battenberg	50	380	apricot	40	300
(per slice: 50 g)	25	190	chocolate	25	300
Carrot	45	400	custard	35	300
(per slice: 50 g)	23	200			
Cheesecake	30	310			
(per slice: 50 g)	15	155	**JAMS AND MARMALADES** (100 g)		
Chelsea bun	55	350	Jam		
(per bun: 75 g)	40	280	fruit	69	260
Cherry	60	400	low sugar	32	123
(per slice: 50 g)	30	200	Marmalade	69	260
Chocolate	60	400			
(per slice: 50 g)	30	200			
Chocolate éclair	35	380	**CEREALS** (100 g)		
(per éclair)	25	270	Bran (natural)	60	270
Christmas	60	320	Bran flakes	70	320
(per slice: 50 g)	30	160	Chocolate rice pops	95	380
Cream bun	25	425	Coco Pops	85	380
(per bun: 50 g)	13	210	Cornflakes	85	360
Crumpet	40	200	Corn Pops	85	380
(per crumpet)	15	80	Crisped rice	90	370
Doughnut			Fibre and fruit flakes	75	350
cream	30	350	Fruit and nut flakes	70	350
iced	45	420	Honey Loops	77	370
sugar	50	340	Honey Puffs	90	390
Fruit	50	320	Honey Nut Cheerios	78	372
(per slice: 50 g)	25	160	Muesli	70	360
Hot cross bun	60	300	Oats, instant	70	370
(per bun: 50 g)	30	150	Porridge oats	73	400
Iced fruit bun	45	300	Sugar-coated cornflakes	90	370
(per bun: 75 g)	33	225	Sugar puffed wheat	85	350
Jam tart	63	390	Sultana bran flakes	20	300
(per tart: 33 g)	21	130			
Lemon curd tart	63	390			
(per tart: 33 g)	21	130	**CHIPS AND CRISPS**		
Lemon tart	33	415	Bombay mix (100 g)	34	544
(per slice: 50 g)	17	208	Dipping chips (100 g)	63	490
Madeira	60	400			
(per slice: 50 g)	30	200	**POTATO CRISPS**		
Marble	60	400	Cheese and onion (100 g)	48	535
(per slice: 50 g)	30	200	(per bag)	12	134
Mini Jaffa cakes	73	398	Potato sticks (100 g)	52	530
(per cake)	5	26	(per bag)	39	400
Sponge			Prawn cocktail (100 g)	49	535
without jam	50	450	(per bag)	12	134
(per slice: 50 g)	25	225	Prawn crackers (100 g)	60	534
with jam	60	350	Pringles Original (100 g)	47	547
(per slice: 50 g)	30	175	Ready salted (100 g)	48	544
Swiss roll	65	350	(per bag)	12	136
(per slice: 50 g)	33	175	Roast beef (100 g)	47	540

Food Item	Carbohydrate (g)	Calories
(per bag)	12	136
Roast chicken (100 g)	46	550
(per bag)	12	140
Salt and vinegar (100 g)	45	550
(per bag)	11	140
Sour cream and onion (100 g)	65	435
(per bag)	14	94
Tomato (100 g)	45	550
(per bag)	12	140

CONFECTIONERY (100 g)
CHOCOLATE

Food Item	Carbohydrate (g)	Calories
Bounty	56	485
Cooking	60	500
Double Decker	65	460
Flake	55	530
Fruit and nut	55	550
Fudge	72	445
Maltesers	61	490
Mars Bar	70	450
Milk	60	520
Milky Way	72	454
Mini eggs	68	495
(per egg)	2	15
Orange	57	530
Ripple	59	528
Yorkie bar	58	526

SWEETS

Food Item	Carbohydrate (g)	Calories
Fudge	80	450
Liquorice	65	280
Strawberry sherbet sweets	93	380
Chewing gum		
sugar-free	<1	40
(per piece)	<1	4
normal – with sugar	30	100
(per piece)	3	10

SUGAR (100 g)

Food Item	Carbohydrate (g)	Calories
Caster	100	400
Demerara	100	394
Granulated	100	400
Icing	100	398

DESSERTS (100 g)

Food Item	Carbohydrate (g)	Calories
Apple pie	30	200
Chocolate mousse	30	225
Lemon mousse	20	185
(light)	20	140
Chocolate sponge pudding	40	210
Christmas pudding	60	340
Creamed rice	17	100
Crème caramel	20	120

Food Item	Carbohydrate (g)	Calories
Custard		
pouring	15	90
powder with full-cream milk	12	100
Ice cream, vanilla	24	190
Lemon meringue pie	40	320
Raspberry mousse	30	245
Strawberry and cream sundae	17	236
Strawberry cream trifle	22	170
Strawberry trifle	18	150
Trifle	30	100

DRINKS

Food Item	Carbohydrate (g)	Calories
Beer (pint)		
ale	16–30	165–320
bitter	14	190
stout	10	200
Cider (pint)		
dry	15	205
sweet	25	240
Milkshakes, thick (per 100 ml)		
chocolate	20	120
strawberry	20	120
Port (50 ml)	6	75
Sherry (50 ml)		
medium	3	60
sweet	4	70

FAST FOOD

Food Item	Carbohydrate (g)	Calories
Bacon and egg muffin (100 g)	25	250
(per muffin)	33	380
Big Mac	44	490
Cheeseburger (100 g)	30	250
(per burger)	33	300
Chicken dippers (100 g)	13	280
(per dipper)	2	50
Chicken, fried (100 g)	25	230
(per piece, approx)	45	420
Chicken McNuggets (per 6)	12	250
(per nugget)	2	42
Chicken nuggets (100 g)	15	125
(per nugget)	3	24
Chips		
fried (100 g)	30	190
oven (100 g)	30	160
takeaway (100 g)	30	240
French Fries		
oven-bake (100 g)	36	240
(per portion)	28	220
takeaway (100 g)	34	280
Hamburger, takeaway		
(per burger)	33	250
Hash brown (100 g)	30	230
(per piece)	15	120

Food Item	Carbohydrate (g)	Calories
McChicken Sandwich		
(per sandwich)	38	375
Onion bhaji (100 g)	16	300
(per bhaji)	4	65
Pizza (all varieties high GI)		
average pizza (100 g)	33	250
(per slice)	25	170
cheese and tomato, deep pan		
(100 g)	45	310
(per slice)	45	310
cheese and tomato, thin		
and crispy (100 g)	28	260
(per slice)	25	230
four cheese, thin and crispy		
(100 g)	32	250
(per slice)	20	155
pepperoni (100 g)	32	267
(per slice)	20	164
vegetable and goat's cheese, thin		
and crispy (100 g)	31	250
(per slice)	21	165
Quarter-pounder (100 g)	20	240
(per burger)	37	420
Saffron rice (100 g)	24	155
Sausage roll (100 g)	25	300
(per roll)	30	370
Spring roll (100 g)	25	230
(per roll)	50	400
Vegetable pakora (100 g)	20	265
(per pakora)	5	60
Vegetable samosa (100 g)	25	225
(per samosa)	7	60

FRUIT

Food Item	Carbohydrate (g)	Calories
Banana	31	125
Mango	20	80

NUTS

Food Item	Carbohydrate (g)	Calories
Cashew	18	570
Chestnut	36	170

PASTA AND NOODLES
PASTA (100 g dry weight)
All varieties including cannelloni, conchiglioni, farfalle, fettuccine, fusilli, gnocchi, lasagne, linguine, pappardelle, penne, rigatoni, spaghetti, tagliatelle and vermicelli

Food Item	Carbohydrate (g)	Calories
	73	360

NOODLES (100 g)

Food Item	Carbohydrate (g)	Calories
Egg noodles	70	340

COMMERCIAL PASTA PRODUCTS (100 g)

Food Item	Carbohydrate (g)	Calories
Macaroni cheese	15	120
Ravioli in tomato sauce	13	73
Spaghetti hoops	12	56
Spaghetti in tomato sauce	13	61

RICE (100 g)

Food Item	Carbohydrate (g)	Calories
Arborio	78	350
Basmati	76	350
Brown	74	349
Thai fragrant	77	350
White rice		
long-grain	76	340
short-grain	78	375
Wholegrain	75	350

SAUCES AND STOCKS
SAUCES

Food Item	Carbohydrate (g)	Calories
Barbecue	65	270
Chilli	50	50
Chutney	55	200
Hoisin	38	180
Horseradish	10	105
HP	27	119
Mango chutney	58	230
Oyster	35	190
Satay	35	450
Seafood	20	335

COMMERCIAL STOCKS
Bisto

Food Item	Carbohydrate (g)	Calories
chicken gravy granules	56	389
original	55	390
vegetarian granules	55	394
Knorr stock cubes		
beef	21	326
chicken	24	301
lamb	16	295
vegetable	22	308
OXO stock cubes		
beef	38	265
chicken	37	243
lamb	43	289
vegetable	42	253

HIGH-GI VEGETABLES

Food Item	Carbohydrate (g)	Calories
Mushrooms, shiitake, dried	64	295
Parsnip	14	65
Potato	16	75
Sweet potato	20	80
Tomato, sun-dried, in oil	25	200

Index

Also available from Vermilion
by Dr Charles Clark

The New High Protein Diet	9780091884260	£7.99
The New High Protein Diet Cookbook	9780091889708	£7.99
The New High Protein Healthy Fast Food Diet	9780091894788	£7.99
The Healthy Low GI Low Carb Diet	9780091902544	£7.99
The Ultimate Diet Counter	9780091889715	£7.99

FREE POSTAGE AND PACKING

Overseas customers allow £2.00 per paperback

ORDER:

BY PHONE: 01624 677237

BY POST: Random House Books
C/o Bookpost, PO Box 29, Douglas, Isle of Man, IM99 1BQ

BY FAX: 01624 670923

BY EMAIL: bookshop@enterprise.net

Cheques (payable to Bookpost) and credit cards accepted

Prices and availability subject to change without notice. Allow 28 days for delivery.
When placing your order, please mention if you do not
wish to receive any additional information.

www.randomhouse.co.uk